Interviewing and Patient Care

THIRD EDITION

ALLEN J. ENELOW, M.D.

SCOTT N. SWISHER, M.D.

New York / Oxford
OXFORD UNIVERSITY PRESS
1986

Oxford University Press

Oxford   New York   Toronto
Delhi   Bombay   Calcutta   Madras   Karachi
Kuala Lumpur   Singapore   Hong Kong   Tokyo
Nairobi   Dar es Salaam   Cape Town
Melbourne   Auckland

and associated companies in
Beirut   Berlin   Ibadan   Nicosia

Published by Oxford University Press, Inc.,
200 Madison Avenue
New York, New York 10016

Library of Congress Cataloging in Publication Data

Enelow, Allen J. (Allen Jay), 1922–
  Interviewing and patient care.

  Includes bibliographies and index.
  1. Physician and patient.   2. Medical history
taking.   3. Interpersonal communication.   I. Swisher,
Scott N., 1918– .   II. Title.   [DNLM: 1. Medical
History Taking.   2. Physician-Patient Relations.
WB 290 E56i]
R727.3.E53   1986   610.69'6   85-7268
ISBN 0-19-503654-9
ISBN 0-19-503655-7 (pbk.)

Printing (last digit):   9   8   7   6   5   4   3   2   1

Printed in the United States of America

PREFACE

The thesis of this book is that interviewing is much more than taking a patient's history. Interviewing is the key to successful clinician-patient relationships. Skillful interviewing makes possible the communication between patient and clinician that fosters a mutually satisfying relationship and leads to the best possible outcome. The interview is of central importance in every stage of continuing patient care from the initial encounter and in every setting in which health care is provided. It is a skill that should be mastered by all health professionals.

This book was written for students of the health professions including nursing, dentistry, medicine, and those students of psychology and social work who plan to make their careers in health care. It is now fourteen years since the publication of the first edition. Changes and additions that went into the second edition reflected talks with students of the health professions who had used the book. In the subsequent seven years, we have learned even more from our students and from other teachers using the book. The third edition thus reflects still further changes including deletions and additions that we believe will further broaden its usefulness. In addition, we have been joined by three collaborators, Lynn S. Baker, M.D., Kenneth Brummel-Smith, M.D., and William F. Skinner, M.D. Their experience in teaching students in Introduction to Medicine and Doctor-Patient Relationship courses made a valuable contribution both to the planning and to the actual writing of this edition of the book.

The key chapter for the student is Chapter 2, on basic interviewing. It presents what might be termed the anatomy of the interview. The general characteristics of open-ended interviewing are given, followed by a detailed description of each of the interview behaviors that makes up the interviewer's repertoire. This knowledge helps the interviewer to choose the action most likely to advance the interview. Many clinicians reduce communication when they ask several questions in a single communication and leave the patient uncertain as to which to respond to. If done repeatedly, it may interfere in the establishment of a relationship of trust and confidence. A clear understanding of the differences among the various interviewer behaviors and of the most likely type of patient response to each will help the interviewer choose the most appropriate one and increase the clarity of his inquiry or other message. As the interviewer strives for a thoughtful, appropriate choice of interview action, his spontaneity may be reduced. This may lead to a certain awkwardness. However, with practice, one's facility rapidly increases and the need to think about each comment is reduced, until open-ended interviewing becomes second nature. Some of the interview behaviors, such as confrontation, are not usually part of one's social communication behavior and must be deliberately practiced with patients if facility is to be acquired.

Asking questions and developing directed lines of inquiry are, of course, essential to diagnostic studies. In Chapter 3, specific attention is given to the skill of asking questions and making inquiries while minimizing the introduction of bias. Included is a section on interviewing patients with communication difficulties, such as the blind or deaf patient.

Chapter 4 describes the patient's emotional responses to interviewing and interviewers. It is best studied after some experience applying the principles described in Chapters 2 and 3. Chapter 5 is a new chapter describing the emotional and behavioral responses of the clinician to illness and to patients. The contribution of

Lynn S. Baker, M.D., is the companion to Chapter 4 and should be studied in conjunction with it.

Dr. Enzer's chapter on interviewing children and parents is unchanged in this edition. Dr. Enzer is both a pediatrician and a child psychiatrist and links the two perspectives.

Two new chapters have been contributed by Kenneth Brummel-Smith, M.D., a teacher of Family Medicine and of Geriatric Medicine. These are the chapters on interviewing the older adult and a revised chapter on interviewing the family.

William F. Skinner, M.D. has contributed a new chapter on interviewing and continuing care, the case examples of which are taken from his own practice of general internal medicine. Chapter 11 is an appropriate continuation of the discussion of the findings and planning of treatment covered in Chapter 10. Thus this book now begins with the initial interview and addresses itself to every stage of continuing patient care.

The first two editions were well received by the students who used them. It is our hope that this third edition is the best of the three and will be even more useful to all students of the health professions.

Santa Monica   A.J.E.
East Lansing   S.N.S.
June 1985

CONTENTS

Interviewing and Patient Care

1

THE INTERVIEW IN CLINICAL MEDICINE

1 INTRODUCTION

Diagnosis and treatment in medicine begin with the interview. Gathering information, evaluating it, discussing the findings with patients, planning, and monitoring treatment all depend on interviewing. The greater the skill of the interviewer, the more complete and reliable will be the information on which he bases his diagnosis. A skilled interviewer will succeed in transmitting findings to the patient so that they are clearly understood, are not unduly frightening, and inspire trust and confidence in the physician. Skilled interviewing affords the possibility of involving the patient in the planning of his treatment, making it much more likely that he will carry out the doctor's recommendations. A good doctor-patient relationship requires effective interviewing and increases the likelihood that the physician will be able to monitor progress in treatment as well as to get early information about developing complications. Finally, good interviewing is the basis of the positive side of health care that is so often sought in vain by patients: that the physician not limit his help to the removal of discomfort but seek to produce a state of comfort and a feeling of well-being. Clinicians are likely to consider the term "medical interview" as synonymous with what is called history-taking. The medical interview is much broader than that.

Failure to follow good interviewing principles will often result in an inaccurate diagnosis or a significant gap in the information needed for planning treatment.

A fifty-three-year-old widow with a long history of anxiety, many somatic complaints without discernable physical basis, and frequent visits to her physician consulted him because of chest pain of several days' duration. As usual, she was quite worried about her new symptom. The physician interviewed her briefly, asking a few highly specific questions. After a somewhat hurried physical examination he noted a slight reduction in blood pressure and assured her. "You're just fine, Mrs. D. We've talked about your worries and fears before. That's all it is." That night she was taken to the hospital by ambulance. She had a myocardial infarction, which was now manifested by severe, crushing chest pain, and a marked drop in blood pressure. Because the range of information elicited during the interview that afternoon was limited, the physician was unable to arrive at an accurate diagnosis.

A thirty-three-year-old divorced secretary with known hypertension was interviewed at a psychosomatic case conference. The Senior Resident in medicine brought her to the conference as a complicated management problem because her blood pressure could not be kept under control with any of the usual anti-hypertensive medications. He had an excellent and detailed account of all of her physical difficulties and the complications of her hypertensions. He described her as a cooperative patient and had found nothing of psychological significance. The interviewer began with an open-ended query: "What kind of troubles are you having?" With great heat the patient replied, "Men!" She went on in a torrent of emotion, sometimes angry, sometimes weeping, to describe difficulties with her employer, her ex-husband, her father, and now with male friends and lovers. She talked about her use of alcohol in large amounts to control her alternating anger and depression. All of this was new information to the resident, who had interviewed her in a highly structured, directive-interrogative manner.

When a patient consults a physician he expects of that physician that he find the sources or causes of discomfort and that measures be taken to remedy the disorder. To accomplish these things, the physician's first task is to gather information upon which to base reasonable hypotheses about the cause or causes of the patient's discomfort. Though the physician has at his disposal a number of methods of obtaining information, some based on observation, others based on instrumentation and laboratory procedures, the most important is the interview.

Interviewing is not, of course, unique to the doctor-patient relationship. It is the most common way of obtaining information to be used by professional persons in their relationships with clients, patients, and applicants. It also plays a role in many social relationships and brief business or professional encounters. Garrett writes:

> Everyone engages in interviewing. Sometimes he interviews; sometimes he is interviewed. The mother interviews the principal of the school in which she is thinking of entering her son. He, in turn, interviews the mother and the boy. Later the boy is interviewed by his prospective employer and, in turn, interviews the latter. Some people because of the nature of their work spend a good deal of time in interviewing. The attendant in an information booth devotes all his working hours to miniature interviews. Lawyers, doctors, nurses, newspapermen, policemen, ministers, counselors, credit men, personnel managers, employers, all devote a considerable amount of time to talking with people, getting information from them, advising them, helping them.[1]

The physician is not the only health professional who uses interviewing to gather data upon which to base clinical decisions. Nor is the dentist. Other members of the health care team are assuming more responsibilities, and interviewing is now used in patient care by all of them. The hospital nurse conducts brief interviews which must be highly focused to collect data so that she can record the patient's physiological and psychological response to treatment. In outpatient health care, nurses and dental hygienists may take initial histories, conduct screening interviews and perform other interviewing tasks. In private offices both may be informal psychotherapists. Social workers and psychologists, members of professions that have traditionally emphasized interviewing skills for data-gathering and counseling, are assuming equally important roles in the health care team. Physician's assistants, nurse-practitioners, and health aides are examples of new health professionals who use interviewing. Since the principles that we are about to discuss in this book apply to all interviewing in the care of patients, we will use the terms "doctor-patient relationship" and "clinician-patient relationship" interchangeably. It should also be noted that when we refer to clinicians as "he," we are conforming to conventional English usage and these pronouns apply to female as well as male clinicians. (We regret that no felicitous alternative is available.)

2   THE ART AND SCIENCE OF THE INTERVIEW

Kahn and Cannell define the interview as a specialized pattern of verbal interaction initiated for a specific purpose and focused on some specific content area, with consequent elimination of extraneous material.[2] This definition, while too broad,* clarifies an important aspect of the clinical interview: the interviewer not only must facilitate communication but at times must guide and even limit it. There are interviewing techniques, used mainly by some mental health professionals, that aim to facilitate communication almost exclusively, making little or no effort to limit it. While this may be necessary in conducting certain, though by no means all, types of psychotherapy, such an approach is inefficient and far too expensive to be generally appropriate in health care. It can be just as inefficient to ask too many highly specific questions early in an interview, as this may cut off communication or limit it prematurely.

In addition to communication skills, interviewing requires an attitude of openness as well as a basic curiosity—a desire to know

---

* Kahn and Cannell's definition could apply to any decision-making conference. It fails to clarify that in a clinical interview one person, the interviewer, has the major responsibility for the outcome. It should also be noted that during any interview the roles of interviewer and interviewee may reverse from time to time for brief or even long periods.

more about a person. The interviewer should have the capacity to transcend any cultural and social barriers between himself and the interviewee so that he can understand what the interviewee means by the words that he uses. And, of course, in medicine successful interviewing requires that the interviewer know enough about the pathophysiology of the illness and its clinical course, as reflected in signs and symptoms, to be able to evaluate the relevance of the information he obtains.

The mixture of art and science of clinical examination upon which the clinical decision-making process rests is nowhere better described than in Feinstein's work *Clinical Judgement.*

> The art of clinical examination comes from attitudes and qualities that are neither obtained nor easily detected by scientific procedures: the clinician's awareness of people and human needs; his ability to temper the rational aspects of his work with a tolerant acceptance of the irrationalities of mankind; his perception of faith, hope, charity, love and other elements of human spirit and human emotion. These properties of care and of compassion, although sometimes dismissed as *merely* "bedside manner," are the fundamental and most important tools of any clinician. With them, he can often give healing or comfort where science fails or does not exist. Without them, his science is unsatisfactory, no matter how excellent.[3]

3 INTERVIEWING IN THE PROCESS OF PATIENT CARE

There is obviously an intimate relationship between interviewing and clinical decision-making. Every interview has the function of collecting information and ultimately leads to a decision. The decision may be simply to do nothing because more information is needed, or it may be highly complex, involving the initiation of a course of therapy. The decision that stems from the interview might be that everything is going as well as could be expected and nothing need be changed. Clinical decision-making is rarely a single, isolated event. Except in those instances when the clinician-patient relationship begins and ends with a single encounter, as in an emergency room or crisis center, decision-making is continuous, both within a given period of illness and over longer periods of time that include episodes of illness and intervals of relatively good health. This is well known to family physicians and those other health professionals who are experienced in continuing medical care. Students and house officers are often far less aware of this and tend to think of a given interview as a complete, self-limiting transaction immediately after which a clinical decision must be made. The fact is that a tentative or preliminary decision might be made, but it is subject to revision with each subsequent interview. The corollary to this is that it is not necessary to gather all of the relevant data in one single interview. The astute clinician knows that he may begin his diagnostic studies with the first interview and that each subsequent interview will add increments of data that will increase the size of his "data bank" about his patient. Also, if the first interview is carried out with appropriate support, in such a way as to increase the patient's trust and confidence as well as his feeling of participation, the interviewer will probably obtain data with greater ease in subsequent encounters with the patient.

There is an often-quoted principle of scientific observation that entering any system or process, either as observer or participant, changes it. The interview has its effect, both on subsequent interviews and on the patient. Attitudes and expectations learned in each encounter have a significant influence on the patient's response to the doctor in the interviews that follow. This is especially true of the first interview that initiates the relationship and, to a lesser extent, of the first in any episode of illness, in a continuing doctor-patient relationship. The clinician who biases his patient's account in the first interview will find that bias clouding his subsequent data and complicating the task of other clinicians who may take part in the patient's care.

In the chapters to follow, we will discuss the interview in data collection and recording, decision-making, and planning and instituting treatment. Interviewing as it pertains to every aspect of patient care is the central theme of this book.

REFERENCES

1. Garrett, A., *Interviewing: Its Principles and Methods.* New York: Family Service Association of America, 1942.
2. Kahn, R. L., and C. F. Cannell, *The Dynamics of Interviewing.* New York: John Wiley & Sons, Inc., 1957.
3. Feinstein, A. R., *Clinical Judgement.* Baltimore: The Williams and Wilkins Co., 1967.

2

BASIC INTERVIEWING

1 THE SOCIAL CONTEXT OF THE INTERVIEW

Each patient and each interviewer has certain expectations for his own and the other's behavior. Some of these are the culturally defined social role behavior of patient and of doctor, nurse, or other health professional. This behavior influences the communication of both parties in the interview and consequently the data, both in form and in content. Other influences on the communication behavior of each include their personal style of communication, family background, socio-economic status, and the ethnic, religious, and other subcultures in which they live or have lived. The interview is also influenced by the physical setting and other aspects of the health care delivery system in which it occurs. All these factors may influence an individual's decision about the person to seek out for health care, the phase of illness in which he seeks help, the type of ailment for which he seeks help, his behavior in the interview, and his response to recommendations and treatment.

The Patient Role

Social role is a concept used by behavioral scientists to describe the patterns of behavior shared by individuals occupying a certain position or fulfilling a certain function in a society. Our behavior varies, to some extent, according to the social context in which it occurs.

We behave differently as we assume the roles of parent, husband, student, worker, poker player, and so on. Conversely, those with whom we interact respond to us differently, depending on how they understand our appropriate role in a given context. That is, they anticipate how we will behave in the social role they attribute to us and respond with this prediction in mind.

The patient usually assumes a sick role before he adopts a patient role. The sick role may be thought of as a deviant role since it prevents the individual from fulfilling some or all of his socially defined functions. This deviant role, however, is usually not morally condemned if it is assumed under the following conditions. First, the incapacity of the individual is considered impossible to overcome by an act of will on his part. Second, the sick person recognizes his deviant state and exhibits a "desire to get well" and to return to social functioning within the limits of his capacity. And third, he expresses this desire by consulting and following the recommendations of a health authority deemed appropriate by others in his social setting. When the incapacity is viewed as caused by the sick person, perhaps through his failure to "take care of himself," he is not accorded exemption from disapproval and often suffers guilt and remorse.[1] This circumstance does not exempt him from the remaining requirements of the sick role; indeed, strict adherence to the treatment regimen may serve as kind of an "expiation" of the "sin" committed against his health.

It is the last aspect of the sick role that brings the patient to the attention of the health professional and forms the core of the patient role. The patient's perception of this role may come from specific instruction in school or by his family, from his previous experience with physicians or other clinicians, from having observed the experiences of his relatives and friends with doctors, or through the portrayal of the doctor-patient relationship in movies, television, and literature. The patient role in our culture is strongly influenced by what health professionals view as appropriate behavior on the part of those seeking their help.

Acceptable role behavior requires of the patient that he "put himself in the hands" of the physician and exhibit "a desire to get well." The patient's behavior will reflect his acceptance of the doctor's authority and his willingness to surrender some of his autonomy. Accordingly, he is usually somewhat passive. He may volunteer information only as encouraged by the doctor to do so, and he may attempt to restrict the information he gives to the general area about which the physician indicates he is interested. The patient is also likely to do whatever he can to keep the level of tension low, that is, to please the doctor. One of the important consequences of the role behavior of patients is the reciprocal effect whereby the physician may inadvertently cut off communication by exerting too much authority and requesting only highly specific information.

The patient will come prepared to speak more freely about his body, his discomforts, and his pain than in other social situations and he will be more reserved in speaking of aspects of life which he considers unrelated to health and illness. Since the patient's role includes compliance with the physician's authority, the patient is usually prepared to accept the doctor's definitions of what is relevant to health and illness and to modify his behavior to meet the physician's expectations.

The Professional Role

Like the patient, the interviewer's behavior in conducting the interview is in many respects a product of his history, his own subcultural reference groups, and his social role. Personal characteristics, including the way he has learned to handle authority throughout his life, will influence his behavior as well as how he and the patient relate to each other. He will tend to behave with the patient as authority figures in the interviewer's life have behaved. His behavior with patients will also reflect the way he has learned to deal with others who were subordinate, weaker, or more helpless than he, such as younger brothers and sisters and younger friends.

Unlike the patient, the interviewer has been trained to subject much of his personal behavior to the professional discipline which governs his conduct in the interview. The medical student, for example, undergoes a long and rigorous socialization process which inculcates in him the appropriate role behavior for a physician in our society. This role includes not only technical skills but a variety of prescribed and proscribed behaviors defining the nature of his relationship to his patients. Other health professionals are subject to similar, though usually less intensive, socialization.

The physician's professional role, including his relative freedom to perform his work without supervision from outside his profession, his position as an arm of the law, for example, with respect to psychiatric and infectious diseases, and the profession's success in enlisting the state to enforce professional standards, enhances the authority of the physician in the interview and influences his behavior accordingly.

2   THE CLINICIAN-PATIENT RELATIONSHIP

What we would term an effective clinician-patient relationship is ideally characterized by trust and confidence in the clinician; a feeling of relative autonomy and appropriate participation on the part of the patient; continuity of the relationship with flexibility in its nature and depth; and reasonable expectations on the part of both doctor and patient.

Trust and Confidence

Illnesses that cause people to seek help are very often accompanied by anxiety, a feeling of helplessness, and disturbances of the relationships between the patient and others around him. Often, too, illness leads to a disruption of family functioning and to loss or threatened loss of income. Therefore, the patient comes to the physician with a characteristic mixture of hope and fear. He hopes that the physician will be able to discover the cause of his discomfort and take appropriate steps to set things right. At the same time, he fears that the physician may not be able to help him and, in some instances, that help is not possible. These fears may be compounded by apprehension over the cost of care or the possibility of painful, disabling, or disfiguring treatment procedures.

Initial trust in the physician's professional skill is usually created by the degree of confidence the physician communicates through his manner and such things as diplomas, certificates, and office atmosphere. It is another thing, however, to have a feeling of personal trust and confidence in the physician. Trust and confidence are built when the physician provides support and when he respects the patient's autonomy. They are also created when the physician (or other clinician) maintains the reserve that defines him as a professional person whose aim is to help, and who seeks no reward from the relationship beyond those given to the professional person for being successful in his work. Of course, previous successful treatment of the patient or his family or friends also provides a basis for trust.

Autonomy and Participation

Three types of doctor-patient relationships have been described by Szasz and Hollender: activity-passivity, guidance-cooperation, and mutual participation.[2] The major variables in the three relationships are the degree of participation and feeling of autonomy on the part of the patient.

In the activity-passivity relationship, the physician uses all of the authority inherent in his status and the patient feels no autonomy, tries hard to please the physician, and does not actively participate in his treatment. While usually required in the management of emergencies, it is the poorest type of relationship for diagnostic interviewing and data-gathering, as well as for much treatment.

In the guidance-cooperation type of doctor-patient relationship, the physician still exercises much authority and the patient is obedient, but the patient has a greater feeling of autonomy and participates somewhat more actively in the relationship. This is more appropriate than the activity-passivity model for a diagnostic interview. But a guidance-cooperation relationship does not encourage emergence of the widest possible range of relevant information. The desire to please the physician still may cause the patient to restrict information to what he perceives is wanted, as well as to bias the information he gives in a direction that seems to be de-

sired by the interviewer. Alertness and great skill in phrasing questions on the part of the interviewer are necessary in order to overcome this tendency. Later in the interview, during the detailed
inquiry commonly called the review of systems, a guidance-cooperation relationship is appropriate.

The mutual participation relationship is the most desirable for
the diagnostic interview, as it is for the management of chronic illness. Here the patient feels some responsibility for a successful outcome, which involves both active participation and a feeling of
relatively great personal autonomy, that is to say, responsibility for
his own behavior. This is created by appropriate moderation of the
physician's use of his authority, a theme that will recur throughout
this chapter. In such a relationship, the widest range of relevant
diagnostic information tends to emerge and the most successful
outcome of treatment is likely to occur. While it is true that some
dependence on the physician is useful, especially in acute and
frightening illness, it is generally not useful to foster the patient's
feeling of dependence. Dependence can reach a point where it
interferes with treatment and prolongs the relationship. The best
clinician-patient relationships encourage the patient to take increasing responsibility for himself at a time and rate consistent with
good treatment.

Continuity and Flexibility

While the clinician-patient relationship ideally has continuity, it is
characteristically flexible in both nature and depth. There are
times when the relationship is intense and involves frequent contacts and detailed explorations of the patient's physical and personal life. At other times the relationship is casual and occasional,
perhaps consisting of an annual checkup or help for a minor and
limited disorder, such as a simple laceration or sprain. The nature
of the relationship may vary from the careful exploration of unex-
plained severe and acute symptoms to counseling, and from routine procedures such as inoculations or superficial examinations to
intensely emotional encounters during times of stress or crisis in
the patient's life. In the most successful clinician-patient relation-

ships a data bank is built through repeated encounters. New information is added as each new problem is explored and its solution sought. The ability to establish this kind of relationship is primarily a function of the emotional and supportive aspects of the interview.

Reasonable Expectations

The patient's expectations from the doctor-patient relationship, and therefore from the interview, are very much influenced by the pain and fear he is experiencing when he consults the doctor. The patient expects to have the source of his disorder found and corrected. He also expects some degree of comforting or care from the physician and some reassurance. His view of a successful outcome of his treatment is that it produce a positive feeling of well-being, not just the absence of pain or discomfort. The fact that this outcome is not always possible is never easily accepted by patients, except for those who are "professional patients," that is, those who have learned to obtain gratification from the sick role. It is important that the physician deal realistically with the patient's expressed and unexpressed expectations from him and from their relationship. Open and frank discussions about prognosis are usually helpful; tact and an understanding of appropriate timing are necessary.

3 THE INTERVIEW MODEL

What kind of interview is most likely to produce a relationship characterized by trust and confidence, an appropriate degree of autonomy and participation, flexibility in its nature and depth, and reasonable expectations on the part of the patient? It is our view that an open-ended interviewing style is most likely to produce the desired type of clinical relationship and to be both effective and efficient in the task of data collection.

Before describing this open-ended model, let us examine two alternative approaches to interviewing. Our observations of physicians in postgraduate courses and of house officers in university hospital clinics led us to conclude that the average medical interviewer is likely to seek information in the most direct manner possible—by asking a great many questions. This style of interviewing might be called directive-interrogative. It is often referred to as history-taking. The physician has a long "list" of items in mind about which he wishes to have information. Each bit of information given to him by the patient is followed by several specific questions elucidating details. In a number of observed situations, certain consistent effects of this interview style were noted. The patient has a tendency to become quite passive. Often the patient makes some early efforts to bring in personal concerns, then ceases the efforts and limits his communication to supplying the information that is being sought. When the interviewer and the patient come from different cultures or different social classes, the patient may struggle to understand the interviewer—with limited success. The interviewer often responds with increasingly specific questions (and sometimes with irritability). The relationship has rarely deepened by the conclusion or the interview. Important diagnostic clues, particularly in the psychological and social areas, may not be picked up.

In the mental health care disciplines, by contrast, one is likely to find very little emphasis on fact-finding through an inquisitory technique and a much greater emphasis on the development of rapport. Much attention is paid to the empathic responses of the interviewer and to the facilitation of communication, and correspondingly less attention is paid to data collection. Facts are not actively sought; they are permitted to emerge. This is especially true of the psychiatric interview that will lead to psychotherapy and of the social worker's casework interview.[3]

The open-ended interview to be described here is a derivative of the interview styles that have emerged in the mental health professions. It has been modified to fit the medical or health care setting. It combines the goals of the fact-finding type of interview with the concern for rapport and the emphasis on emergence of information, rather than the extraction of facts, that characterize the interviewing style of most mental health professionals. The description of the characteristics of the open-ended interview and the most likely responses of patients to the interview behaviors of the physician are based on five years of research in interviewing, using an interaction analysis scale developed by Adler and Enelow.[4, 5, 6] The guiding principle of the open-ended interview is that the clinician should exert the least amount of authority necessary to obtain the information he is seeking within the time allotted for the interview.

There are four general characteristics of this style of interviewing. First, the interview should be carried out in an atmosphere that encourages spontaneous behavior on the part of the patient. Second, the interviewer's behavior should encourage communication. Third, the interviewer should give attention to the patient's non-verbal behavior as well as his story. Fourth, the interviewer's specific information-seeking actions should be those that exercise the least control first and the highest degree of control as late in the interview as possible.[7]

The Interview Setting Should Be Optimal

An atmosphere that encourages spontaneous behavior has both physical and emotional attributes. Comfort and privacy should be provided whenever possible. The interviewer should arrange for the fewest possible interruptions.

The private physician conducts most extensive medical interviews in his office, his most congenial environment. It is here that he feels most at home and where, consequently, his most spontaneous behavior is likely to occur. Both the doctor's and the patient's behavior will be influenced by the way the office is used. Both can communicate more freely if the setting of the interview is a quiet consulting room, with reasonably comfortable furniture, and if there are few or no interruptions. While it is perhaps easiest to secure the conditions for a successful interview in the physician's office, it does not necessarily follow that these conditions will exist. Many physicians permit the telephone and office personnel to interrupt their interviews, do not allow sufficient time for the interview, or narrowly limit the topics discussed. Some physicians make a practice of conducting interviews in their examining rooms, where the patient is partially clothed or under a drape sheet on the examining table. The patient rarely feels at ease under such circumstances. He is likely to feel both powerless and self-estranged without the clothing which announces his identity to others and confirms it for himself. The social distance between the doctor and the patient is likely to be increased. Docility, obedience, embarrassment, and efforts to please the physician will reduce the amount of information from the patient and sometimes bias it.

The least suitable setting for an outpatient interview is probably the clinic of a large public hospital. The physical setting is often uncomfortable and unattractive, and it is likely to afford little privacy. The clinician is usually on a tight time schedule. Both the clinician and the patient are frequently caught in a maze of bureaucratic procedures, and often both are aware that the patient will see a different clinician on his next visit. The interview can bring together a clinician and patient of quite different socio-cultural backgrounds, with the many attendant difficulties. All this creates problems that require a great effort on the interviewer's part if they are to be overcome.

The immediate situation provided in a hospital is likely to be unfavorable for an effective interview. The patient is more frequently than not in a ward or shared room, and hospital personnel or visitors may interrupt the interview. The patient is usually in bed, while the interviewer is clothed and mobile. In this situation, some interviewers stand at the foot of the bed, some at the side of the bed, and some sit on or near the bed while talking to the patient. In each case, the effect on the interview varies. The physical distance from the patient has an effect on the emotional distance; they vary directly with each other. The standing physician speaking with a patient who is lying down creates a status difference that reduces communication. The physician who is sitting and close enough to touch the patient will be helping to create an atmosphere that is supportive and that encourages communication.

The interviewer's behavior should encourage communication.

The interviewer should communicate by his manner that the patient can respond freely and discuss whatever he wishes. As a rule of thumb, the fewer the clinician's utterances to keep the patient talking, the better. This is especially true in the earlier part of the interview.

The interviewer should give attention to the patient's non-verbal behavior as well as his story.

Non-verbal communication is often more indicative of a patient's inner state than his verbal account. Information not contained in words may be clearly expressed in behavior, manner, and appearance. An important way of facilitating the patient's spontaneous account is to call his attention to the observed behavior.

The interviewer should move through a cycle of information-seeking behavior that begins with low use of authority and proceeds to progressively greater use of authority.

The interview is best begun with a broad, open-ended question such as "What kind of difficulties are you having?" As the patient answers, the interviewer should encourage spontaneous elaboration on his account through facilitating remarks and gestures. If the interviewer observes that that patient is encountering difficulty in describing his problems or discomfort, or if it is difficult to understand his account, he should point it out to the patient. If there is incongruity between the patient's behavior and his account, the patient's attention should be drawn to the observed behavior. Lastly, if these methods have not yielded specific items of needed information, or provided information at that point in the interview where specific details are needed to fill in the story, the interviewer should use direct questions.

The principle is this: spontaneous reporting tends to produce the broadest range of information, most of which is likely to be relevant. When verbal communication ceases, non-verbal communication continues. Pointing out the non-verbal behavior tends to encourage the verbal expression of the inner experience. For example, a patient who is told that he has a worried and pained look may then describe his chronic low-grade neck stiffness and headache. Feelings, such as sadness or fear, may be first expressed after the non-verbal (behavioral) evidence has been brought to his attention. If this does not succeed, questioning may be necessary. If the patient can express himself well, very few questions may be necessary. A very important reason for limiting the interviewer's control over the patient's communication is to minimize bias in the information offered. The wording, timing, and sequence of questions, as well as non-verbal behavior accompanying them, all may provide cues that influence the patient's replies.

4 BASIC INTERVIEWING TECHNIQUES

Opening the Interview

The open-ended question, such as, "What kind of troubles have you been having?" says to the patient, "I am interested in anything you may feel is important enough to you to tell me." In return interviews, an appropriate variant might be, "How have you been getting along?" Interviewers who do not use the open-ended question frequently close off whole avenues of important information since they do not give the patient permission to develop areas not covered by the interviewer. Yet some patients, especially children and adolescents but also adults, are unable to respond to an open-ended question with a detailed account. In such a case the interviewer may be tempted to begin direct questioning at once. If the sole reply to "What kind of troubles have you been having?" is "Well, I've been having a lot of headaches," followed by silence, the clinician may fall into the trap of asking a series of questions like, "How long have you had them?", "How long do they last?", "Where does the pain seem to be?", "What relieves them?", and so on. Each specific question the doctor asks will increase the probability that the patient will give the exact information requested and lapse into silence, awaiting the next question.

Before embarking on a line of direct, specific questioning, the interviewer should try less controlling actions. These include silence, facilitation, and, if appropriate, confrontation.

Silence

The least controlling thing an interviewer can do is to be silent and "give the patient the floor." If the patient falls silent, the interviewer should consider being silent himself for at least a brief time. Ordinarily the patient will soon feel free to resume his account. That the clinician is not speaking does not mean that he is not communicating. His facial expression, posture, and movements all tell the patient something about the interviewer's response to his account and to him as a person. An attentive facial expression and posture tell the patient non-verbally that he has an interested listener. On the other hand, standing over a bed patient suggests that you will not remain long enough for him to tell you very much. It is a good idea to look at the patient but not stare continuously into the patient's eyes. Looking distracted, fidgeting, slumping in an attitude of fatigue, looking away from the patient, and examining the chart all indicate that the interviewer's attention is not fully focused on the patient. This non-verbal message will inhibit the patient considerably.

Thus, while the patient is communicating freely about important matters, the doctor's behavior of choice is an interested, attentive, and relaxed silence. Whether to remain silent or to speak when the patient falls silent is a choice which requires the skill that comes with experience. During an interview silences of only a few seconds often seem interminably long. Silence is frequently quite uncomfortable for the inexperienced interviewer. The busy practitioner is also likely to tolerate silences poorly because of his schedule consciousness. A common response of both beginning and busy practitioners is to search for a question or a remark to keep the conversation going. But one can learn to tolerate silences through practice. This is a worthwhile exercise, for there are times when it is very useful to the interview for the clinician to maintain his silence after the patient has stopped speaking.

One of these times is when the patient has stopped speaking in order to clarify his thoughts, to recollect facts, or to find a way of adequately expressing something. The patient may explain such silences with remarks like, "Let me think a minute," or "How can I say that better?" This kind of thoughtful silence is rarely accompanied by signs of increased tension. The perceptive interviewer can usually recognize this situation and wait for the patient to continue. An interruption may make it more difficult for the patient to express himself clearly.

Another situation requiring a decision either to remain silent or to initiate some action occurs when the patient appears to have said all he wants to say and has come to a natural pause. The pause may be signaled by a remark and by the patient's demeanor, indicating that he has finished and is waiting to hear from you. The best choice at this juncture depends on a number of circumstances.

First, the clinician should consider how often these pauses have been occurring and how lengthy and complete the patient's narrative has been. If the patient has been limiting his remarks to a few phrases or sentences and then waiting for you to take the initiative again, you may have been interrogating him. If you have been asking a great many direct questions and continuing after brief replies, the patient will assume that brief replies in response to your questions are what you wish and expect. If, upon reflection, you feel you have placed yourself in such a situation, a pause on your part may encourage the patient to go on. If the patient continues to remain silent, it may be helpful to try a comment or facilitation with a relatively low level of control.

If, after reflecting on the course of the interview, you realize that you have been working hard to help the patient tell his story on his own, and you sense that the patient is "holding back" and that his non-verbal behavior reflects tension or discomfort, your silence is again likely to be appropriate: in the silence which follows, the patient's discomfort may well increase, and he may then tell you on his own what is bothering him and give you an opportunity to deal with it. This could be something in the immediate environment, such as telephone interruptions, the intrusion of office personnel, or a feeling that you are uninterested. On the other hand, it may be reticence, shame, or embarrassment about telling important parts of his story. The difficulty in communication which has developed may also be due to the patient's discomfort in speaking freely to someone of a different sex, age, class, race, or ethnic background. The patient may fear the possible diagnosis and react to this anxiety by failing to communicate freely in order to "ward off" the knowledge that he has the disease he dreads. Or his discomfort may be related to important events or circumstances in his personal life that you need to know about in order to manage the patient's treatment successfully. Whatever the reason for his evasiveness and discomfort, a pause will allow his discomfort to become clearly evident to both of you. If he does not speak about it spontaneously, you are ready to point out the difficulties in communicating which you have been observing. A confrontation in this situation will frequently result in a discussion of the difficulty the patient is encountering. This will usually permit the interview to proceed smoothly.

The situation in which a patient has been communicating freely but shows increasing difficulty with a particular topic and halts the account is another instance of silence best handled by remaining silent. In the ensuing pause, the emotional basis for the failure of communication may become apparent, and the clinician can then proceed with a confrontation leading to a discussion of the difficulty.

There is one time when it is mandatory for the clinician to remain silent. This is when the patient has stopped speaking because he is overwhelmed, or about to be overwhelmed, by emotion. Sometimes one may forestall or attenuate an expression of strong emotion—most frequently weeping—by prematurely saying something to the patient, thereby failing to reduce the patient's tension. There are several reasons for remaining silent until the patient has expressed strong emotion and brought his feelings under control. Foremost is the fact that open expression of feelings is almost always therapeutic for a patient. In addition, it is likely that a patient will be able to express himself more adequately after a release of emotion. He may well be able to speak of things which he could not bring himself to discuss before. If, on the other hand, the patient decides to control himself and withhold his feelings, he has the opportunity to do so. He makes the choice himself; it is not forced on him.

The extent to which the patient is helped and the interview is facilitated by permitting a display of feeling depends very much on what the doctor says and does after it has subsided. A supportive response is almost always helpful. This will be taken up later in this chapter.

In some cases it will not be appropriate for you to remain silent when a patient pauses. If an overly talkative patient who has been dominating the interview and preventing the efficient gathering of diagnostic information stops talking, for example, you might take the opportunity to obtain some of the information you need. Another time that you would not necessarily remain silent at the patient's pause would be when you felt a need for clarification of what the patient had been saying. There are several ways you might choose to proceed, these will be described later.

In the early part of an interview, silence may allow the patient to go on to a new topic. If the patient shows signs of increasing tension as a silence develops, one can acknowledge what was just said, ask a broad question concerning this or other problems the patient may have, or comment on the patient's discomfort. Near the close of the interview, when the interviewer feels he has a generally complete account of the patient's situation, he may not pause but instead immediately move to obtain some specific information with questions.

There are a few "don'ts" with regard to the use of silence on the part of interviewer. Most individuals in our society are made uncomfortable by long silences in ordinary conversation. A doctor who overuses silence may be perceived by the patient as cold or distant. Certain individuals, particularly adolescents, do not tolerate silence well. When the interviewer perceives that his silence produces discomfort in his patient to the point of reducing further communication, he should become more active.

Facilitation

Encouraging communication by manner, gesture, or words that do not specify the kind of information sought is called facilitation. It represents a greater use of authority than silence but still exerts a low degree of control. Since a completely impassive silence on the part of the interviewer is relatively uncommon, silence and facilitation tend to go hand in hand. An interested, attentive manner is, of course, facilitating. Any change of facial expression or posture displaying greater interest or attention is a facilitation. A common mode of facilitation is a nod of the head, conveying, "I'm listening," "I understand what you're saying," or "Go on." This message is encouraging to the patient but can be overused. Inexperienced interviewers frequently relieve their own tension during the interview with what might be called the "head-nodding syndrome." The clinician should also take pains not to nod his head for facilitating purposes when the patient has been expressing a strong opinion. In such instances, his action may be mistaken for approval or agreement.

A similar message is conveyed to the patient with an occasional "mmm-mmm" or by postural shifts toward the patient or into a position of greater alertness. The doctor may also interject short words or phrases such as "yes" or "I see" without interrupting the flow of the patient's narrative.

Another type of message that is facilitating is the action that conveys "I don't understand." This may be non-verbal, such as a puzzled look, or a verbal statement of confusion on the order of "I don't follow you" or "I'm sorry, but I don't understand."

When a patient has stopped or appears to be about to stop discussing a topic and the interviewer wants more information, he also may encourage the patient to continue by repeating his last few words. This may be done with the inflection of a question or merely as a repetition. For example, either "the last few days" or "the last few days?" will invite the patient to continue. Another verbal facilitation is a brief summary of what the patient has been saying. This indicates that you have understood him and are interested in further information. A brief summarizing remark will usually encourage the patient to continue, without explicitly directing him to do so or specifying what subject he should discuss.

Facilitation can also be used to return the patient to a topic previously introduced. This is done by referring back to a phrase previously used by the patient which indicates the matter of interest to the clinician. For example, in the course of describing her child's respiratory complaints, a mother may mention that her child has had a fever and then go on without elaborating. After she has completed her description, the physician can then say, "You say Johnny has had some fever?"

Facilitation, then, evokes communication by suggesting to the patient that the doctor is interested in what the patient is saying and is encouraging him to continue. It may also suggest, but not require, that the patient explain or expand on something he has said. A good interviewer with a normally communicative patient should be able to gain much of the information he needs by attentive silence and facilitation. When the doctor senses that the patient is not speaking freely and clearly, however, he should consider making a confrontation.

Confrontation

In confrontation the interviewer describes to the patient something striking about his verbal or non-verbal behavior. Here the clinician exerts a little more control over the interview than he does in facilitation. Facilitation is a suggestion to the patient that he elaborate on a topic he has introduced. Confrontation directs the patient's attention to something that he may not be aware of or, at best, be only dimly aware of. As a result, a confrontation very often has the effect of introducing a new topic. Examples of confrontations are: "You look sad," "You seem frightened," "You sound angry," "I notice that you have been rubbing the back of your neck."

Like permitting a silence, confrontation poses a difficult problem for the beginning student of interviewing. Students are often self-conscious about using it. In ordinary, casual social conversation one does not call the attention of the person with whom one is talking to striking aspects of his manner or behavior of which he is probably unaware. To do so would usually be considered impolite. Very often, too, confrontation is a hostile act; frequently it is used in heated controversies. Since confrontation is not part of one's ordinary repertoire of social behaviors, one must develop through practice its use as an effective expression of sympathy or support during an interview.

One situation in which a confrontation is useful has been previously alluded to, namely, when the interviewer observes that the patient is having difficulty in providing information. Some of the possible reasons for this have already been discussed. It was suggested that if there is a pause during which the patient's discomfort has become evident and, perhaps, its nature revealed, a confrontation is in order unless the patient ends the silence by describing his difficulties. The form of the confrontation will depend on what the doctor has observed. Often useful are such comments as, "You seem to be having a good deal of difficulty telling me about this" and, "You appear quite uncomfortable." The patient who gives brief answers without elaborating may respond to, "I notice you say very little except when I ask you questions." A common response is "Oh, I didn't know you wanted me to go on."

Note that the above confrontations describe how the patient appears to the interviewer. They are based on what he has *observed*. They do not make inferences about the patient's motives or his specific emotional state. It is, of course, possible that the interviewer has been incorrect in ascribing discomfort to the patient. In this case the remark will give the patient an opportunity to explain the difference between the clinician's perception of his behavior and his own. Such an explanation usually provides useful information.

The confrontation is not formulated as a question. At first glance, it might seem more efficient to ask, "Why are you uncomfortable?" or, "Why do you have so little to say?" There are several reasons for avoiding such questions. First, they assume that the physician is correct. A question puts more pressure on the patient to agree with the doctor than a mere statement of the doctor's observation. Second, a direct question also requires that the patient make some reply. The patient may not have developed sufficient trust in the doctor to reveal the required information. He may make an evasive, partial, or even a false reply. Third, the patient may not know or be able to formulate the answer to the question. Feeling forced to reply, he gives a misleading or uninformative answer. The question "Why?" asks for a causal explanation. Many persons, especially among the lower socio-economic classes and the culturally deprived, do not think in terms of intra-

psychic causes for their behavior or problems, and this is the realm
of causation to which the doctor is usually referring. Even more
important, a complete response to such a question would require
the patient to discuss his genetic endowment, his socialization
from infancy to the present, the set of circumstances under which
he is living, and what is happening in the interview situation. Asking why allows the patient to select some plausible "cause" out of
that part of these data which are available to him. His explanation
may very well be what he thinks the clinician believes or wishes to
hear. This often leads to mutual acceptance of an explanation
which appears plausible to the interviewer but which may or may
not be either accurate or valid. In pointing out the patient's communicative difficulties the doctor is attempting less to discover
their causes than to permit the patient to express the feelings he
is then having. This expression may be sufficient in itself to permit the patient to continue; if not, the doctor may be able to assist
the patient in continuing once he has listened to this expression.

Another situation in which confrontation is useful occurs when
the patient's non-verbal behavior communicates something to the
interviewer that the patient is not talking about. For example, a
housewife may be describing some set of physical symptoms, and
her doctor observes her dejected posture, her sad look about the
eyes, her low and monotonous voice, and her twisting fingers. By
some remark like, "It strikes me that you look very sad," the doctor
responds to her non-verbal rather than her verbal communication.
Slightly reddened eyes or trembling of the chin or lips may indicate that the patient is on the verge of tears. A sympathetic confrontation such as, "You look as if you are about to cry" may offer
the patient an opportunity to give vent to her feelings of despair
by open weeping. This may have a most valuable therapeutic
effect. Physicians in particular tend to avoid situations that encourage a patient to cry for fear the patient will later be ashamed
or embarrassed about it. This fear very often stems from the doctor's own feelings about the shamefulness of crying. If the doctor
responds to the weeping patient tactfully, it is very unlikely that
the patient will feel ashamed or embarrassed.

It is appropriate, too, to confront a patient when his voice, posture, bodily movement, or facial expression betray emotions such as anger or anxiety. One can say, "I get the impression that you are angry," or, "You sound angry." To an anxious patient one can say, "You look worried," or, "You seem tense," or one can remark on the behavior which betrays tension or anxiety by saying such things as, "I notice you're chain-smoking," or, "You're trembling." All such remarks tend to evoke a freer expression of feelings from the patient. Valuable information is derived and other needed information can be obtained more expeditiously after the patient's expression of his despair, fear, anger, or other strong feeling. Lastly, if the clinician handles the situation sensitively, the patient will feel increased trust and confidence.

A particularly appropriate time to confront a patient is when his verbal and non-verbal behavior are clearly incongruous. For example, a patient may speak about very sad things in an indifferent manner, about insults or gross injustice without displaying anger, or about comfortable circumstances and happy events in a mood of dejection. A comment on these discrepancies may lead to valuable information about the patient's difficulties and especially about his conflicts.

A confrontation is also appropriate when there are inconsistencies in the patient's story. This almost always leads to valuable information.

There are a few cautions to be stated about confrontations. In ordinary conversation, when we speak of confronting someone we often mean a hostile accusation. This term often has an unpleasant and unnecessary connotation of anger, even though there are many types of helpful and positive confrontations. When confrontations are made in an interview they should reflect sympathetic interest in the patient. Sometimes the interviewer's irritation with some behavior of the patient may be the cue that calls this behavior to his attention, but it is his interest in this peculiarity of behavior and in furthering the goals of the interview that should prompt and be expressed in the confrontation. A second caution concerns the overuse of confrontation. Even though the patient is confronted in a sympathetic manner, he may feel criticized if he is confronted too often. Confrontations can develop a nagging quality. No more than one or two confrontations about the same or related observations are appropriate in any interview.

Questions

The question, which could be called directive evocation[8] requests information and specifies the area of information desired in the response. This is the highest use of authority and it exercises the greatest degree of control thus far discussed. Open-ended questions vary in the degree of authority they represent, depending on how closely they specify the area in which the reply is expected.

Questions that require a very specific answer are rarely appropriate if the interviewer does not know how he will use the information in arriving at a decision. If direct questions are properly phrased, answers will most often be brief but high in information content.

Even greater control is exerted when the question is so phrased that a yes or no answer is called for. A similar form is the multiple choice query in which the interviewer specifies a list of specific replies he expects the patient to choose from: "Does this pain come on before, after, or during meals?" These two types of questions we may term *checklist questions*, since they verbally offer the kind of question which may be answered by checking off a pre-printed response on a questionnaire.

Checklist questions are generally to be avoided in an interview. Both types tend to stop the interchange. The patient "checks off" the reply and waits for the next question. Furthermore, both types tend to suggest that the interviewer is not interested in information which does not fall into the categories provided and expects the patient to "pigeonhole" his reply categorically. More communicative patients may overcome this suggestion and provide relevant information not requested, but the interviewer should not rely on this when formulating questions. It is particularly difficult to create good multiple choice questions spontaneously. The categories should be exhaustive and mutually exclusive. If all possible alternatives are not offered, bias is introduced. If all alternatives are presented, the question is likely to be so complex that it confuses the patient. Multiple choice questions are, therefore, best given in written form. Questions represent the interviewing behavior most likely to produce biased information. A discussion of ways to avoid bias will be found in Chapter 3.

At what points in the interview is it wise to use direct questions? The first is anytime one cannot get needed information with a lower degree of authority. The second is when the broad outlines of the story have emerged and specific information about details is needed. These include the review of systems, inquiry into past illnesses, and parts of the mental status examination. Chapter 3 will deal with these aspects of the interview.

Direction, the highest use of control, refers to statements or actions that indicate, instruct, or demand of the other what he should do in such a way that an expected compliance is clearly indicated. Directions to speak, such as, "Tell me more about that," exert the full force of the doctor's authority. However, the direction cited does not limit the range of information that the patient will give to anything like the degree that a direct and highly specific question will. Thus, directions, too, can allow a patient considerable latitude in what he says, though little latitude in the topic he speaks about.

Somewhat less control than with either questions or directions is exercised when the interviewer makes a *suggestion.* A suggestion is a subtle direction or advice which may guide the patient's thinking or behavior. Because of the authority of the clinician, it will have much more effect on the patient than the same words would have in a different setting. For this reason, suggestion is the commonest way of biasing information. This can be done in several ways. One is by the wording of the question. Another is by shifting topics, which may say to the patient, "That's not important— no more about that." It can also be done by interpreting what the patient has said, or by mentioning a tentative diagnosis. Suggesting a pattern of pain or a symptom must be avoided in diagnostic interviewing. However, suggestion may be helpful in treatment; it is probably the basis of the placebo effect.

Support and Reassurance

In the first part of this chapter, we mentioned that trust and confidence in the clinician is built when, among other things, the patient is offered support. This is also true of reassurance when appropriate and correctly timed. The clinician's ability to be properly supportive and reassuring helps create an atmosphere in which the patient is encouraged to communicate. It also helps to promote the continuity of the relationship.

Support refers to any act which communicates the interviewer's interest in, liking for, or understanding of the patient, or which promotes a feeling of security in the relationship. Examples of supportive statements are, "I understand" and "That must have been very upsetting." A summary that conveys a sympathetic comprehension of what the patient has just said is supportive.

One of the most important times to express support is after the patient has expressed strong feeling. After a confrontation to which the patient has responded with weeping, or the expression of hitherto tightly controlled fear or anger, support is most important. It increases the solidarity of the relationship and helps the patient to continue his account.

It must be clearly understood that supportive words without a supportive attitude on the part of the interviewer will sound hollow and will fail to accomplish their intended purpose. Without a genuine interest in the patient, a feeling of friendliness, and a desire to be helpful, supportive words are simply not supportive.

Reassurance includes words or acts which tend in the direction of restoring the patient's sense of well-being, worthiness, or confidence. When patients are very frightened, a reassuring remark may have a remarkably helpful effect. As with support, if the words are reassuring but the clinician's attitude does not convey reassurance, the attempt will fail. To be effective, reassurance must be based on evidence or fact and be genuine. Cliches are rarely reassuring.

Since reassurance depends on acceptance of the doctor's authority, reassurance should not be given in a way that creates unreasonable expectations. Staying close to fact is the best way of avoiding this. The clinician can reassure by citing what he has learned up to that point and how it can be interpreted. On the other hand, stating, "Everything will be all right," or, "There is nothing to fear," unless the evidence clearly supports such a statement, is a poor use of reassurance. The statement "You are making satisfactory progress" is reassuring only if it is based on good evidence that the patient can understand.

5 NON-VERBAL COMMUNICATION

Throughout the interview, when the patient is speaking or silent he communicates simultaneously at two levels. One level, the more obvious verbal or lexical communication, has so far been the primary focus of this chapter. The other, usually referred to as non-verbal communication, has been popularized as "body language."

An early systematic study of body language was made by Charles Darwin, who in 1872 published *The Expression of the Emotions in Man and Animals*.[9] Darwin studied the behavior, posture, and facial expressions that accompany emotional states. He viewed them as involuntary, instinctive communications that can be easily understood. Weeping, for example, has a communication function, that of summoning help. He studied the non-verbal accompaniments of such emotions as anxiety, grief, and despair and used photographs to illustrate his contention that these facial expressions serve as universally understood non-verbal signals.

In addition to these psycho-biologically determined expressions which appear to be universal, many non-spoken communications of emotions, including gestures, inarticulate sounds, facial expressions, and body movements, are learned at an early age by those who share a given culture. Such communications may be thought of as having a vocabulary consisting of gestures with specific meanings. Even the space a person places between himself and another and the way he uses time (in the sense of lateness or promptness or speed of movement) have meaning or communications. Hall[10] calls this "the silent language."

How may this silent language be perceived in the data-gathering process of the interview? Since data about the emotional status of the patient can be obtained from both verbal and non-verbal behavior, it is as important as the patient's verbal account. At times, non-verbal behavior is essential to understanding what the patient is trying to say. Obtaining it requires that the interviewer carefully observe the patient's behavior—including gait, demeanor, posture, facial expression, and tone of voice—throughout the interview and during the physical examination. Taking notes and looking at one's chart or clipboard while writing is a common barrier to "reading" body language. Even more frequent, however, is the simple failure to observe the patient carefully and to heed the communication that is not being provided in words. This may happen because many clinicians are less comfortable with the patient's feelings than they are with "facts," such as descriptions of symptoms, dates, and times of onset. Anger, sadness, resentment, and fear are also facts, but some clinicians prefer not to deal with them. Yet they may be as relevant to an understanding of the clinical problem as the more "objective" data.

Some signals may appear in the words used by the patient. For example, a recurrent allusion to something that is never further explained may mean the patient is leaving out something significant. In this case, one might inquire about it using either an open-ended question or a confrontation.

> The patient, very tense while telling his story, alluded to the various physicians he had previously consulted as either trustworthy or not. Thus, he would say, "Then I went to see Dr. Jones. I trusted him," or "I was sent to Dr. Smith. I didn't trust him." The interviewer commented, "I notice that you mention whether or not you trust each physcian you refer to." (Confrontation) After a moment's silence, the patient said, "I guess that's a real problem with me." This led to a description of a disturbing experience with a brusque physician several years earlier, after which the patient developed an attitude of suspicion toward all physicians. Having explained this, the patient visibly relaxed. Further interviewing clarified that distrust of persons in authority was a factor in the patient's general tension and anxiety.

When a patient uses one word or phrase repeatedly it often signals an important preoccuaption. A discreet inquiry may bring out feelings of worry, despair, depression, or anxiety.

Facial Expressions

Sadness is often mirrored in the face of the depressed patient. A downturned mouth, lackluster eyes, or a slight quivering at the point of the chin or lower lip are signs of depression. Clenched teeth with bulging masseters indicate tension, sometimes due to anger. A fixed smile implies that the patient is anxious to please you and may be fearful. Sometimes a forced smile is used to mask depression and to fight off a desire to weep. Simply pointing out the smile may help the patient clarify the underlying meaning. Anxiety usually shows in a patient's face as a discernible look of apprehension, often accompanied by rapid, shallow breathing. The apprehensive patient often has darting eye movements, looking about the room and usually not maintaining eye contact except for brief periods. Physical pain can be communicated through facial expressions, even when the patient is not fully conscious.[11]

A person's eyes can be quite revealing. Depression shows there. Eye contact that is too intense may occur when the patient glares at the interviewer (anger) or attempts to be seductive (manipulative behavior), expressions which, of course, are not difficult to tell apart. Inability to maintain eye contact may reflect guilt feelings, as when a guilt-laden topic is being discussed. It may also indicate anxiety or the patient's difficulty in coping with his feelings about the interviewer. Normally, when patients are listening carefully or are intent on telling their story, they will look directly at the interviewer but will not appear apprehensive or angry unless those feelings are being immediately experienced in response to what is being discussed. They will not, however, give an impression of staring at the interviewer.

Posture

The patient's posture communicates something of his attitude toward you, usually his dominant emotion. Posture can reflect openness (relaxed arms at sides, slightly slouched in the chair) or a closed, defensive, distrustful attitude (arms closed, hugging one-self, sitting up very straight). Slumped shoulders and a bowed head are marks of depression. Anxiety is often signaled by the patient's shifting about, finger tapping, foot and leg movements, or gripping the arms of a chair with white knuckles.

Note whether the patient leans away from you or shifts his chair to increase the distance (thereby indicating defensiveness or distrust) or leans toward you or moves closer (thus expressing a desire for more intimacy). There are also ethnic differences in the distance from others that one finds comfortable. For example, people from Latin cultures may move closer to you than Anglo-Saxons do.

If a patient's posture reveals belligerence, this attitude must be dealt with, as it can be a deterrent to a successful interview. It is best to call attention to it in a tactful, non-threatening way so that it can be brought out into the open and discussed.

The patient was a forty-three-year-old construction worker being seen for evaluation in the Rehabilitation Medicine Clinic. The interviewer noticed that the patient's fists were clenched, his jaws tightly clenched, and that he sat stiffly erect. The interviewer said, "I can't help but notice how you are sitting. You look like you don't want to be here." "I don't," said the patient, and went on to describe, with considerable anger, the great number of examinations he had had and his feeling that he was considered to be either a hypochondriac or a malingerer. After the interviewer reassured him that he held no such attitude and that the ultimate purpose of the interview was to initiate treatment, the patient relaxed and the interview proceeded uneventfully.

Tone of Voice

We all know that the same words spoken in two different tones of voice may have very different meanings. If asked how one's day has been, a reply of "Just fine," said in a warm and pleasant tone usually means just that; the same words said quickly, tonelessly, and without conviction may really mean, "Don't bother me. I've had a bad day and I don't want to talk about it." When interview-

ing a patient, especially on follow-up visits or after an interval of
some length since the previous interview, the response to the usual
inquiry about how the patient has been feeling may be just such a
brief comment. The intonation of the words may then be the clue
to how the patient feels. It may also indicate the patient's attitude
toward the interviewer or the need for further encounters with
health care providers. The interviewer's response is usually keyed
more to the non-verbal communication of the patient's tone of
voice than to the content of the words. Alertness to the intonation
and a simple comment or query about it may open up a whole
vein of useful information.

Gestures

Valuable information about the patient's feelings can be obtained
by observing his gestures. These are often involuntary and probably instinctive, though how pronounced and expressive they are
is influenced by the culture from which the patient comes. Covering the eyes or mouth may mean, "I don't want to see it" or "I
don't want to talk." Reaching out to put a hand on the interviewer's
arm or to finger his coat lapel may mean, "Listen to me" or "Pay
more attention to me." Shrugs, waggling the palm of the hand, or
holding the palm outward toward the interviewer are easily read
messages that usually emphasize the speaker's words or can substi-
tute for a verbal message. When a patient rubs or repeatedly
touches a part of his body, one should comment on or inquire
about it. The motion usually means pain or discomfort in that
area. Anxiety is often signaled by gestures such as rubbing the
chin, pulling at the lip, twisting fingers, or tapping fingers or feet.
A typical gesture of the frightened, guilt-ridden, or worried person
is the partial elevation of one shoulder or the arm as though preparing to ward off a blow.

Congruence

Any non-verbal message from the patient that suggests something
other than the content of the verbal message or seems to be in

conflict with it should be given special attention. As we have said, gestures, facial expressions, posture, and tone of voice are more reliable indicators of feelings and attitudes than words. Since verbal messages are under conscious control, they are subject to censorship and may be used for purposes of persuasion, to mislead others, or to hide facts one does not wish to reveal. But body language is not so easily censored and will usually give reliable indications of the patient's emotional state. Lack of congruence between verbal and non-verbal messages may indicate that something is being omitted, whether deliberately or unconsciously. Thus, the skilled interviewer who notes a discrepancy between the verbal and non-verbal messages will inquire about it. An effective way of doing this is through confrontation. For example, "You know, Mr. Smith, you say you feel just fine but you look very unhappy." This will frequently focus the patient's attention on his mood. Much new information may then emerge. When patients have difficulty facing certain problems and are attempting to keep their concerns out of their consciousness, their words may serve to help them do that. Their involuntary body expressions will help you decipher the hidden message and bring the patients to an awareness of problems for which there may be some treatment.

The open-ended interview, in summary, represents a style of interviewing that adds features of the interviewing approaches characteristic of psychiatric and social casework to the traditional medical interview. The medical interview emphasizes data collection and aims for high efficiency in gathering detailed data within limited time periods. The aspects added from mental health interviewing include greater attention to rapport and to the development of the clinician-patient relationship and an attempt to facilitate the *emergence* of facts rather than their *extraction* from the patient, thereby creating the opportunity for less biased and more relevant information, both verbal and non-verbal. It relies on a differential use of the clinician's authority, never using more authority than is required to get the needed data, and on the ability of the interviewer, through appropriate support and reassurance, to express his interest in helping the patient.

6 AN EXAMPLE OF AN INITIAL DIAGNOSTIC INTERVIEW

The following interview was tape-recorded at a teaching confer-ence. The patient, a forty-eight-year-old married woman, was in a wheelchair. The marked deformity of her hands was characteristic of advanced rheumatoid arthritis. She was smiling in a forced and unconvincing manner that contrasted markedly with her sunken and weary-looking eyes. Her face and the angle of her shoulders communicated depression, as did her tone of voice.

The interviewer introduced himself and the students present. The interview then proceeded as follows:

DOCTOR: What kind of troubles are you having? [facilitation]

PATIENT: (*quietly*) I come to orthopedic clinic for joint injections.

DOCTOR: For joint injections. I see. Can you tell me about that? [facilitation]

PATIENT: To reduce the pain and keep the stiffness down, that's all that keeps me going . . . (*her voice trails off*)

DOCTOR: (*repeats softly and thoughtfully*) That's all . . . [facilita-tion]

PATIENT: (*her voice picks up in volume*) That keeps me going, that's all that has for the last four years, that keeps me able to do what little of my housework that I do, and take care of myself and get around what little I do. If I don't get them, I am practically down because the pain gets terrific and I haven't the willpower, let's say, after this many years to make them bend against the pain. I proba-bly could bend them if I tried hard enough, but I have too many of them now.

DOCTOR: Too many of them? [facilitation]

PATIENT: Too many joints affected. Before, when the pain was con-fined to my arms and my legs, it wasn't in my neck and hips.

DOCTOR: (*takes patient's hand*) May I see your fingers there? They are sort of swollen and kind of spindle-shaped. And you have trouble bending them here? Right? (*demonstrating for the class; direction*)

PATIENT: More so there. (*points to another joint*)

DOCTOR: I see. You say you've been getting these injections for four years, but I would suspect you've had the trouble longer than that. [support; confrontation]

PATIENT: (*voice drops again. The words sound weary and toneless*) I have had it fourteen years. Just this month I have had it fourteen years.

DOCTOR: (*slight surprise*) Just this month? How do you remember with such accuracy exactly when it began? [question]

PATIENT: (*emphatically*) Wouldn't you if you went to bed one night all right and couldn't get out of bed the next morning? You wouldn't forget.

DOCTOR: (*sympathetically*) It was that sudden. [support]

PATIENT: (*stridency disappears from voice*) I mean, of course, we know it was working on me. I mean, it stands to reason, but I had no symptoms of any kind, I never was sick. I had thyroid surgery when I was seventeen and had a couple of babies and outside of that I was the healthiest person that ever was, as far as outward appearance was concerned. And I felt fine. Then, like I say, I just did a normal day's work one day and the next morning I couldn't get out of bed. But I slept through it, that's the amazing part of it. Nothing awakened me. I went to bed around midnight and as always I got up at six o'clock. When the alarm went off, I couldn't even turn over. My feet were all swollen, and my hands were just like that (*holds up her hands*). The pain was terrific. Of course I was petrified. I had no idea what in the world was the matter with me. I mean, I had never heard of arthritis except in people that were older. My grandmother complained of arthritis in her knees a little bit when she was about eighty years old but that was what I associated with arthritis. I didn't dream of it, I thought of everything else. I wondered, did I have polio, or what did I have? I just, I mean . . .

DOCTOR: (*interrupts*) How old were you? [question]

PATIENT: Well, I would be . . . I will be forty-nine in July. I was thirty-four, and thirty-five in a couple of months.

DOCTOR: (*repeats softly to encourage patient to resume flow of narrative*) You went to bed one night, and the next morning couldn't turn over. [facilitation]

PATIENT: (*sadly*) That's right. I couldn't dress my children, cook meals, dress myself, or anything. It was sort of a problem. We'd only been out here a short time then. We came out in December from back East and this hit in May, so I mean I didn't know too many people. It was rather a difficult situation. But then I mean I got to where I could get around better, but it was after some

months. I still couldn't bend my hands enough to feed myself or
to dress myself in July. And that I can remember because I had a
son killed that July, so I remember at that time I couldn't comb
my hair or feed myself; so, it was probably, oh, about September
before my hands really got to where I could grasp things and
know I was going to hang on to them, and to button buttons and
comb your hair and do things that you normally would do. They
looked anything but normal, but I mean I could bend them. I had
a peculiar color to my skin. It was real yellow, almost like a person
that had jaundice, real slick and shiny. My whole body was that
way. That's one thing I do remember.

DOCTOR: You remember it all with a great deal of clarity, don't you?
[confrontation]

PATIENT: (*reflectively*) Well, I've been studying this thing for a good
many years trying to think of, going through everything that I can
think of, trying to think of something that might give the doctors
an inkling of what would help me. After all, I laughed at the doctors when they said that if I didn't go to the doctor I would get
down. I didn't think the doctor knew what he was talking about.
I thought if you kept walking and going to the things I had always
gone to, that you wouldn't get stiff. I just couldn't believe it. When
it happened it was rather a shock.

DOCTOR: When it happened? [facilitation]

PATIENT: After I had this first attack I got better for a while. I was
taking my son to the doctor. The doctor wanted to talk to me about
my arthritis but I wouldn't let him. I said that I wouldn't get down
because I just knew I wouldn't. Of course, I wouldn't accept it in
the first place. I guess that's probably been my downfall. I fought
it all the way. I was a little independent, let us say. Never had to
ask anybody for anything before. But now I do, I'm afraid. I guess
I do, much to my dismay.

DOCTOR: You say you were kind of an independent person? [facilita-
tion]

PATIENT: (*with pride*) Well, what I mean is I've always done for myself, and I like to do for others and I like to do things for myself.
I don't want to ask other people to take me here or do this for me.
Like a lot of people. This sounds silly in a conversation like this,
but I have friends that say: "Oh, won't you pin up my hair for
me?" That sort of thing. Well, there's nothing physically wrong
with them. They could do it themselves.

DOCTOR: But you were never like that? [facilitation]

PATIENT: (*emphatically*) No, I wasn't.

DOCTOR: You sound sort of proud of yourself about that. [confrontation]

PATIENT: (*hastily*) Well, no, I didn't mean to sound that way. What I meant was I just . . . well, I don't know how else to express only I just like to be on my own.

DOCTOR: You must have been a hardworking person then, because you said that when this happened, you went to bed at twelve, which was your customary time, and got up at six. [confrontation]

PATIENT: Actually, I mean, well if you want . . . do you want what I did the day before it happened? It was just a routine day. Probably I did washing. I don't actually remember that. I cleaned up the house because I was going to have guests for dinner. The carpenter had built on a new room, so I, my younger son and I, had gone outside and hauled wheelbarrows of dirt and cleaned up all the mess that the carpenter had left and put in flower beds and . . .

DOCTOR: And you said that was just an ordinary day? [confrontation]

PATIENT: (*with hesitation—slightly flustered*) No, but I mean I was by . . . I never was one that . . . I mean, I just always was active.

DOCTOR: Back East too? [facilitation]

PATIENT: (*with evident pride*) Well, I sort of had to. I mean I was the oldest of the children in our family, and my Dad wasn't well, and I worked out when I was still in high school. After I had this thyroid surgery and got settled down again, why, I wouldn't go back to school because they had to take me out of school in the middle of my junior year, and I was too . . . my pride again. I wouldn't go back in a small town and graduate. My class had already graduated so I worked, oh, for a year or two, and helped my brother and sister get clothes and books so they could go to school. And then I was fortunate enough to have somebody that was interested enough in me to see that I did go on to school. They offered me a chance to work for my room and board, so therefore I went to a town where there was a teacher's college and went to high school and took college work and worked for my room and board. And, may I say, *I worked*. Not like they do now. I worked in the days when they didn't give their dinner parties in hotels and such, and you did all the cooking and all the dishes. And I mean that was the type of homes you worked in. Besides that, I carried five subjects. Besides that, I made good grades, but I studied until three o'clock in the morning.

DOCTOR: You said this was a teachers' college. You became a teacher? [question]

PATIENT: Well, no, that wasn't my ultimate aim, although I ended up getting married. I suppose you know. I worked long enough to get my teacher's certificate and then turned around and got married, but what I wanted to do was teach for a few years and then go to designing school in Chicago. But I mean I had a purpose in mind when I went there. That was the only way I knew that I was going to get money to do what I wanted to do, because I had to finance myself.

DOCTOR: I see. But you turned around and got married? [facilitation]

PATIENT: (*flatly*) Yes sir, and then went on working.

DOCTOR: Looking after a family? [question]

PATIENT: Well, no. I had to work to support us. I didn't have a family until I was . . . let me see, our first son was born in 1940, and I was married in 1934.

DOCTOR: That seems like a long lag. [confrontation]

PATIENT: Well, to be right honest with you, I wanted a family. But there for a time I tried and lost it.

DOCTOR: You kept miscarrying? [facilitation]

PATIENT: I finally just put myself in bed and had one. I stayed sort of, let us say, not so active. I managed to get two that way. That was the end of my family.

DOCTOR: You stopped at two? [facilitation]

PATIENT: Well, I stopped at two. The doctor wanted me to have more after we lost our other son. But my husband wanted to know who was going to take care of them with me like this.

DOCTOR: After you lost your other son, you mean shortly after . . . [facilitation]

PATIENT: (*interrupts*) Um hmmm, I mean after I had this we lost our youngest son, and so I did want to have another one because I don't approve of raising one by themselves. But we didn't due to this arthritis, and I guess maybe it was wise because I would have tried, and maybe it would have been a little difficult, perhaps.

DOCTOR: Have you been continually disabled since you, since it started in the last fourteen years or has it come and gone? [question]

PATIENT: (*bitterly*) It has never come and gone. It has gotten progressively worse. Little by little, more joints were affected, the pain was worse, more deterioration of joints, degeneration, or whatever you want to call it, of the bones. Then I guess every time that I did feel a little good, why I would try to make up for what I hadn't done before. So I probably defeated the doctors in many of their attempts to help me, and I had quite a few doctors who have been very kind to me and very interested in my case. But I did too much, like the first time they gave me cortisone and I thought, this is it. I have it licked. For a month, I did.

DOCTOR: When was that? [question]

PATIENT: Well, when they first released cortisone to physicians to use. I think, November 1950.

DOCTOR: I see. That's when they started you on it? [facilitation]

PATIENT: They started it by injection. Gee, it worked beautifully. (*her eyes light up momentarily*) I had no pain. I really felt like I had found the answer. But I soon found out I hadn't. (*sadness returns*)

DOCTOR: You soon found out you hadn't? [facilitation]

PATIENT: But I guess those two months of being able to do things and get around was probably worth it. I don't know. Worth the price of cortisone in more ways than one, because I know I did a lot of joint damage while I was taking it because I couldn't get settled down. I just didn't sleep. I mean, I was just constantly on the go, trying to catch up and do all the things I hadn't been able to do for a few years. So that's why I say unknowingly I defeated the thing that might have helped me. Another time was when they put me in braces. And again I thought I had it, and I really got along beautifully. People felt sorry for me, but their sympathy they could have saved, because I felt, what a relief to be able to get around. But I wore them from about 1954 to the latter part of 1957, about November. Then this hip went bad and I just couldn't take the pain anymore.

DOCTOR: Now, were you on cortisone all that while? [question]

PATIENT: (*with feeling*) Oh, no, no, no.

DOCTOR: You went back off it again. [facilitation]

PATIENT: Oh, they only . . . I only took cortisone for those two months of 1950 and then again in October of 1957. That was when my hip got so bad. But it made me so unsettled. I couldn't sleep or stop doing things and moving around.

DOCTOR: You're not on it now? [question]

PATIENT: (*emphatically*) Oh, no, I don't want to ever be on it again.

DOCTOR: You know, I noticed something about you, that you smile a great deal. [confrontation]

PATIENT: (*in a self-satisfied tone*) Well, I've always been happy.

DOCTOR: Always? You don't ever get down? [question]

PATIENT: Oh, yes, I do. The past few years since this thing has been with me, and my leg just won't take it, and I can't do very much with my hands. I have quite a few spells of depression and my age is beginning to catch up with me. Since last September I've noticed it a lot . . . more depressed, and I don't have the outlook that I did. I sort of, I keep slipping. I haven't found anything to hang on to. You know, to look forward to. And then this elbow got real bad in February, and I couldn't use my arm, and Dr. L. put it in a cast, and I was in that for two months, and he thought perhaps he'd operate on it and fuse it in a position like this. That was the way I had the cast on. The pain was so much less. So that has kind of fallen through because the bone appears to be bad. They don't know if it will hold, so you see it doesn't give you much to look forward to. If I could think of some way to get this bone started being something again. But when it's that way you wonder, what about my legs and hips—how long are they going to hold up?

DOCTOR: You know, I have the impression that you sort of keep smiling as though this would somehow, this would really keep you from feeling depressed. [interpretation]

PATIENT: (*slightly embarrassed*) Gee, I don't know. Ask anybody that has known me for years . . . I mean that's been the comment I've had ever since I can remember, that I smile a lot.

DOCTOR: That you smile a lot? But, you see, your eyes aren't smiling, just your mouth [confrontation]

PATIENT: (*tears come to her eyes, smile vanishes*) Now, yes. That's one thing the doctor has always said about me. My eyes, they never showed that I had been sick or had pain or anything until just in the last few years. Now they have gotten blah with the inside of me. Before they weren't like that. (*weeps*)

DOCTOR: (*after a period of silence*) Well, it was very kind of you to come here and submit yourself to this interview. I can see that it has been difficult for you. [support]

PATIENT: Well, if I can be of any help, why, I'm glad to do it.

DOCTOR: You have been. Thank you very much.

Discussion

In any interview, the interplay between doctor and patient primarily determines what data will emerge, what aspects of the patient's story will be told. The interviewer who wishes to get the most informative behavioral picture will strive to create an atmosphere that encourages this. In the foregoing interview, this process is initiated by an open-ended question, which allows the patient the freedom to define the problem in any terms she wishes. (*"What kind of troubles are you having?"*)

The patient initially characterizes her "troubles" by referring to the type of treatment she receives. When the doctor seeks clarification, she not only identifies her symptoms but also provides a clue to the central role treatment plays in her life. (*"That's all that keeps me going."*) As the doctor listens to these opening responses, he must make a decision, as must be done frequently during an interview. With what aspect of the patient's behavior should he concern himself? A rule of thumb is that the clinician should address himself to that quality of the communication which seems to be more important and immediate to the patient.

In this interview, the depressive tone of the patient's opening remarks stands out and tells him much more than the words. To facilitate the communication of her feelings, the interviewer therefore repeats a few words of the last sentence (*"That's all . . ."*). Encouraged by this, the patient proceeds to elaborate on her medical history, and in describing the struggle with her illness, she conveys a feeling of weariness and defeat. At this point, the interviewer turns his attention to the deformity and limitation of movement, partly for his own information and partly to demonstrate both to the class.

After obtaining this information, the interviewer encourages the patient to continue her story. The questions do not change the direction of this narrative, although the interviewer, picking up on previous information, asks for some details about the length of illness. The questions are aimed at helping the patient enlarge on what she has already said. At this point the patient surprises the doctor with one of her statements. (*"Just this month I have had it for fourteen years."*) His reaction expresses his feeling that it would be unusual after fourteen years to remember the month an illness began. The patient responds with considerable feeling as she justifies the reasons for her clear memory of the event. (*"Wouldn't you if you went to bed one night all right and couldn't get out of bed the next morning? You wouldn't forget."*) The physician's supportive and sympathetic tone of voice, as well as the content of his comment (*"It was that sudden"*), encourages her to continue her account of that period. It is important to remember that when the patient perceives a supportive attitude on the part of the physician, the desire to confide in him grows.

As the patient describes the sudden onset of her first major attack of rheumatoid arthritis, the interviewer interrupts briefly to establish the patient's age at that time. Immediately after ascertaining this, he reestablishes the continuity of the patient's narrative by repeating her last words before the interruption. One could justifiably criticize this interruption as unnecessary, since a basic rule of interviewing is not to interrupt the progress of the patient's narrative by asking for information. In this instance, the same information could have been obtained later. The risk of shutting off Mrs. K. was minimized by immediately shifting back to the theme, thus permitting her to pursue her story.

The patient now provides an increasingly vivid description of the progress of her illness. She inserts, without pause, a reference to a tragedy in her life—her son's death. The physician may decide to explore this at some point and clarify its role in the patient's situation, but inquiries now would break into her story and interfere with its development. At this point, all we know is that her son died, that she briefly mentions it without visible feeling, and that the event and the arthritic symptoms are associated in her mind.

The doctor is struck by the detailed quality of her account and comments on it. (*"You remember it all with a great deal of clarity, don't you?"*) The response to this confrontation reflects the patient's attitude toward illness—apparently an obsessive preoccupation. In addition, it reveals that she is not a passive observer of her

illness. (". . . *trying to think of something that might give the doctors an inkling of what would help me.*") Rather, she feels she must "help" the doctors cure her illness. This attitude will be seen to have a great deal of importance as the interview proceeds.

The patient also gives a very clear picture of how she responded to the doctor when the original diagnosis of arthritis was made. ("*I didn't think the doctor knew what he was talking about.*") She was unwilling to face the diagnosis ("*The doctor wanted to talk to me about my arthritis but I wouldn't let him*"), and it becomes evident that management was probably complicated by her refusal to accept a medical judgment, which she accomplished by actively blocking communication. But real events made it impossible for her to maintain this defensive attitude. ("*When it happened it was rather a shock.*") Through facilitation ("*When it happened?*") the doctor encourages her to explain what the shock was, and as she does so, it becomes clearer why she resorted to denial. She prizes self-sufficiency and independence so highly that when faced with conditions that prevent this kind of behavior, she cannot accept them. ("*I don't want to ask other people to take me here or do this for me.*")

Mrs. K.'s need to feel independent should play an important role in her medical management. Rheumatoid arthritis can be an extremely crippling disease in its later stages, so that severe limitations are placed on the capacity to look after oneself. For a patient who values hard work and independence as much as Mrs. K. does, psychological care will be essential. Promoting communication will help reduce her tension, which in turn may have some effect on her physical status. While the evidence at this point is not at hand, it is a reasonable hypothesis that this patient feels guilty about not contributing usefully to her family. She should be given an opportunity to discuss the rationality of these feelings.

At this point, another facet of her self-concept appears: her pride in being a hard worker. However, she cannot accept the doctor's confrontation ("*You sound sort of proud of yourself about that*"), for in her system of values conscious boasting about virtues would be viewed as a failing. She immediately disclaims pride.

("*Well, no, I didn't mean to sound that way.*") When the doctor confronts her in another way ("*You must have been a hard working person, then*"), she describes an enormously productive day, indicating how she values hard work. The story of that day probably has gotten better and better during the fourteen years that have ensued, especially during the recent years of enforced idleness spent in a wheelchair.

The interviewer now confronts the patient with her assertion that the herculean labors of that last day were characteristic of her life before the illness. ("*And you said that was just an ordinary day?*") Of course, this is highly unlikely. But it brings out clearly how a formerly active patient, now confined by physical illness, views with nostalgic pride the days of productivity and independence that are forever behind her.

The patient observes that she had always been active. This provides an opportunity for the doctor to fill in more past history. The next question ("*Back East too?*") is keyed to what the patient has been discussing at this point and therefore does not really change the subject. Instead, it is a request for further information on the same topics—self-sufficiency and hard work—that the patient has been discussing.

In response to this question, the patient tells how she was forced to become independent early because she was the oldest child in the family and because her father was ill. At this point, there is no mention of her mother, which is a significant omission of a traditionally protective figure. However, there is the first clear indication that she must have been lonely or had a feeling of emotional abandonment. ("*And then I was fortunate enough to have somebody that was interested enough in me to see that I did go on to school.*") The theme of work and accomplishment is extended, and an emphasis on intellectual endeavor appears. It is pertinent to note the contrast in the patient's narrative between her role as a household drudge and the pursuit of pleasure she observed in those around her. This suggests that her enforced independence at an early age and sense of abandonment could be a source of anger.

The picture that is developing is that of a driven, compulsive, overly controlled woman. The patient now adds another significant bit of information which the interviewer identifies as a means of expanding the past history. (*"You became a teacher?"*) The patient reveals that she had a specific ambition and a plan. Her desire to become a designer also gives us a clue to a creative, artistic side of her personality. With this apparent goal within reach, however, she obliterates it by putting herself in a position where further schooling is not possible because she must work to support herself. The patient keeps herself in the same bind that has characterized her whole life. The interviewer has now elicited one of the most significant characteristics of the neurotic personality: the tendency to repeat ineffective and even irrational methods of solving problems.

At this point, the interviewer decides to investigate the new, though related, theme of her marriage. However, he commits a common error in interviewing. The question he asks (*"Looking after a family?"*) is putting words in her mouth. As so often happens, he learns that he has jumped to an inaccurate conclusion. She talks about her childbearing history, and a whole vein of information about her early marital relationship is closed off.

The patient describes her difficulty in carrying a child to term, which must have been a source of considerable emotional distress. The fact that she had to accept a passive role during pregnancy must have been difficult for her. (*"I stayed sort of, let us say, not so active."*) It now becomes clear that her childbearing history is related to the course of the rheumatoid arthritis. The patient has come back to her physical condition, so the doctor now finds it appropriate to fill in further history concerning the arthritis.

As the patient provides more details on her arthritis, her strong commitment to duty is underscored by the observation that whenever there was even slight improvement, she would work very hard for a while. (*"Then I guess every time that I did feel a little good, why, I would try to make up for what I hadn't done before."*) A likely reason for this, indicated earlier, is a sense of guilt about neglecting her family which goads her on. But there is also a note of regret that her activities nullified the doctor's efforts. (*"So I prob-*

*ably defeated the doctors in many of their attempts to help me,
and I had quite a few doctors who have been very kind to me and
very interested in my case."*) The concern shown by some physicians in her case was presumably important to her. For a woman
who probably felt emotionally abandoned in early life, the doctor-
patient relationship may have been a vehicle for satisfying emotional needs. The management of such a relationship can be quite
complicated. An overly solicitous or protective attitude on the
physician's part can reinforce neurotic reactions to illness.

In describing her feelings of guilt about not being a more compliant patient, she introduces an important piece of medical information, namely, her treatment with steroids. Together with the
specifically medical information, the doctor learns something of
the emotional impact of steroid therapy on the patient. Her hopes
were raised high and then dashed by a transitory positive response
to cortisone.

Her restless over-activity and sleeplessness suggest a rather frequent complication that occurs when steroids are administered. It
is common to see mild euphoria, over-activity, talkativeness, rest-
lessness, and insomnia in patients receiving steroids. The picture
can resemble hypomania, and in some patients it may develop the
intensity of a full-blown manic psychosis. In such patients, sudden
withdrawal of the steroids may precipitate a severe depression.
When steroids produce the symptom picture of a manic attack,
they should be withdrawn gradually.

The patient again suggests that her behavior may have contributed directly to this deterioration in her condition. (*"I mean, I
was just constantly on the go, trying to catch up and do all the
things I hadn't been able to do for a few years. So that's why I say
unknowingly I defeated the thing that might have helped me."*)
She has emphasized this point several times, so that self-blame and
guilt increasingly appear as important factors in her emotional picture. In the management of this case the doctor is going to have to
discuss the past with her and clarify that she probably was not de-
feating the medical attempts to help her.

With a fairly complete history of the rheumatoid arthritis, the interviewer decides to shift his focus to a direct exploration of the patient's mood by directing her attention to her behavior. He has been aware of a fixed, unconvincing smile on the patient's face. The smile is conveyed only by her mouth, not her eyes. By drawing the patient's attention to what her facial expression communicates, he hopes to bring more of her feeling to verbal expression. This is undertaken in two stages. The first is to comment on the smile; the second will be to call attention to her eyes. The patient begins to talk about the depression she feels. (*"I don't have the outlook that I did."*) Her concept of an independent role has probably included a feeling that it is always necessary to remain optimistic and to make others feel that this has been her unflagging attitude. So it may be hypothesized that she did not permit herself to burden others with her problems. But old patterns of adjustment are deteriorating, and there are no new ones available to her. (*"I sort of, I keep slipping, I haven't found anything to hang on to."*) In situations like this, a psycho-therapeutic relationship may be especially useful in facilitating the development of new attitudes and in helping patients come to terms with reality.

What the patient is saying is clearly depressive in character. Instead of commenting on the content, however, the doctor emphasizes the incongruity between her unhappy thoughts and her appearance of cheerfulness by making an interpretive comment about the fixed smile. (*"You know, I have the impression that you sort of keep smiling as though this would somehow, this would really keep you from feeling depressed."*) In effect, he is probing to determine if the patient consciously and deliberately strives to hide her depression. But she evades this by saying that people have always noticed how much she smiles.

The interviewer then completes the confrontation, calling attention to the look in her eyes. This has the effect of bringing her feelings into full expression. (*"Now they have gotten blah with the inside of me."*) She weeps openly. This makes clear that the depression was not far below the surface. After expressing emotion with open weeping, a patient usually feels a sense of relief.

The patient's closing remark indicates how important it is to her to feel useful. (*"Well, if I can be of any help, why, I'm glad to do it."*) The implication for her management is clear. In addition to physical therapy, and in keeping with her degree of disability, she needs some kind of meaningful work to do. This will help combat depression by diminishing her preoccupation with herself and elevating her self-esteem.

At this point, the doctor brings the interview to a close. She has wept, has had an opportunity to recover, and shows a feeling of relief. If this were not a demonstration, the interviewer would have encouraged further expression of her feelings and then followed this with questions, including a review of systems. This was precluded by time constraints.

This clinical example illustrates how an interview was handled so that the patient's depression, which she has habitually concealed would emerge. An awareness of this depression in a compulsive worker, driven to feel productive and useful, was essential in planning the management of her case.

REFERENCES

1. Parsons, T., *The Social System.* New York: The Free Press, 1951.
2. Hollender, M. H., *The Psychology of Medical Practice.* Philadelphia: W. B. Saunders, 1958.
3. Gill, M., R. Newman, and F. C. Redlich, *The Initial Interview in Psychiatric Practice.* New York: International Universities Press, 1954.
4. Enelow, A. J., L. M. Adler, and P. Manning, "A Supervised Psychotherapy Course for Practicing Physicians," *Journal of Medical Education,* 39, 140-46, 1964.
5. Adler, L. M., and A. J. Enelow, "A Scale to Measure Psychotherapy Interactions." Paper read at the annual meeting of the American Psychiatric Association, May 8, 1964, Los Angeles, California.
6. Adler, L. M., and A. J. Enelow, "An Instrument To Measure Skill in Diagnostic Interviewing: A Teaching and Evaluation Tool," *Journal of Medical Education,* 41:281-288, 1966.
7. Payne, S. L., *The Art of Asking Questions.* Princeton, N.J.: Princeton University Press, 1951.

8. Enelow, A. J., and M. Wexler, *Psychiatry in the Practice of Medicine*. New York: Oxford University Press, 1966.
9. Darwin, Charles, *The Expression of the Emotions in Man and Animals*. Chicago: The University of Chicago Press, 1965.
10. Hall, Edward T., *The Silent Language*. Garden City, N.Y.: Doubleday and Co., Inc., 1959.
11. DiMatteo, M. R., and Friedman, H., *Social Psychology and Medicine*. Amherst, Mass.: Delgeshlager, Gunn & Heath, 1982.

3

OBTAINING ADDITIONAL SPECIFIC INFORMATION

Four classes of information need to be explored in every medical interview:[1] biological, psychological, social, and cultural. *Biological information* generally reflects the pathological changes induced by the disease process as they influence the patient's functioning and subjective sensations. This is obtained during the interview itself, as well as by physical examination and laboratory testing. *Psychological information* reflects the personality of the individual who is experiencing the disease process. This is obtained by careful listening and observation throughout the course of the interview, and is specifically sought during the mental status examination. *Social and cultural information* reflect the environment in which the patient has developed his illness. They include the patient's socio-economic status, level of education, employment history, family structure and stability, and ethnic and religious group. All of these external variables can have a significant impact on the patient's health, his desire to seek medical attention, and his ability to utilize treatment recommendations.

While much of this information may be spontaneously provided by the patient, it is frequently necessary for the clinician to intervene to obtain specific information about a problem that has been tentatively identified. This may require asking direct questions. As we previously noted, interviewers often resort to direct questions too early in the course of the interview. Physicians, in particular, tend to have difficulty refraining from prematurely testing a possible diagnosis suggested by a problem cue. By asking questions too early in the course of the interview, the physician easily destroys the patient's initiative in telling his story. A great deal of specific information can be obtained from the patient's spontaneous account, making it possible to ask fewer highly directive questions with their resultant constriction of range of information. Direct questions can then be used to fill in the gaps.

1   QUESTIONING DURING THE OPEN-ENDED PHASE OF THE INTERVIEW

While direct questioning of the patient should usually occur only after the patient seems to have completed telling his own story spontaneously, direct questioning may be indicated much earlier with the patient who rambles and reiterates or strays away repeatedly into unrelated or unimportant topics. Questions which seek clarification of topics the patient has just volunteered—such as the precise time sequence of events, the exact location of a described phenomenon, the exact amount of a drug taken; and similar questions—will usually be well tolerated during a patient's spontaneous account if they do not interrupt him and are introduced at an appropriate pause. Such questions may heighten his responsiveness and increase his efforts to be precise if they can be seen as evidence of the physician's interest in gathering all relevant data.

A word of caution is in order here. Questioning for clarification and to add significant details can shut off communication if it is directed to a topic about which the patient is defensive or has a great deal of conflict. If the interviewer feels that a given topic may be such a conflict-laden area, it is best to save that detailed inquiry for a later point in the interview. This is wise for several reasons. For one, it permits the patient to develop some feeling of trust in the interviewer, if he is able to. For another, it avoids a possible premature cessation of all communication, as occurred in the following example:

A student was interviewing a patient who had been admitted to the hospital because of severe chest pain that was thought to be a possible myocardial infarction. The patient had a long history of frequent attacks of angina pectoris. During the spontaneous account of his difficulties, the patient said he had been taking 5 or 6 nitroglycerine tablets daily and frequently took Demerol tablets. At an appropriate pause, the student began an inquiry into the frequency with which he took Demerol, the dose, and so forth. At first the patient supplied the information; then, visibly stiffening, he ceased to do so. He asked the student to terminate the interview, stating, "You're asking me too many questions."

2   AVOIDING BIAS IN DIRECT INQUIRY

Regardless of the time or reason for introducing direct questions, good interviewing technique requires that direct inquiry be conducted in a manner which does not bias the resulting communication. The principle is this: accuracy in communication is facilitated when the interviewer does not suggest responses he expects or approves of by the wording of his questions or by his demeanor, tone of voice, or other non-verbal communication. The interviewer's manner can be a source of bias. Facial expressions or gestures which convey moral approval or disapproval, surprise, or greatly accentuated interest or attention will influence what the patient tells or does not tell. The wording of the interviewer's communication can also reveal his own biases and thereby influence the patient's account.

Designers of public opinion surveys have made a careful study of ways of avoiding bias in wording questions.[2] One of these is to avoid emotionally loaded words. For example, "Is she a good baby?" is less likely to elicit accurate information than "How often does the baby cry?" "Have you ever had a pregnancy terminated?" is preferable to "Have you ever had an abortion?"

In general, the more open-ended the question, the more likely the answer will be accurate. It is best to begin direct questioning with general questions and then gradually move to more specific, detailed questions, a process called *narrowing*.[3] Ask "When does the pain come on?" before asking "Does the pain come on right after meals?"

As the interviewer seeks more detailed information, it becomes increasingly difficult to formulate open-ended questions. Therefore, as questions become highly specific, alternatives should be stated. From behavioral science research on question wording, it has been learned that a question like "Does the pain come on right after meals?" will elicit more "yes" responses than will a question like "Does the pain come on right after meals, or do you notice it at other times?" In so wording a question, one should give each alternative equal weight, as in "Does exertion bring on the pain, or do you notice it at times when you have not been exerting yourself?" Even adding "or not?" to a single alternative will reduce the likelihood of a biased response to some degree.

It is most important to formulate questions in a way that does not suggest an expected answer or pattern of pain. Thus, "Does the pain stay in one place or does it move or travel?" is a good question. "Does the pain shoot down your leg?" is more likely to bias the patient's account. Confrontation may be used to avoid the introduction of bias. For example, if a patient repeatedly rubs some part of his body, such as his knee, it is better to use confrontation, such as "I notice that you're rubbing your knee," than to ask, "Does your knee hurt?"

Another point at which there is danger of introducing bias is when facilitating the patient's communication by summarizing what he has just said. Here one may unthinkingly introduce an inference about what he has said, or reflect a personal judgment about it, either critical or approving.

The timing of questions and of shifts in topics can also introduce bias. It is important, therefore, to avoid interpretations or suggestions about the nature of the problem during information-gathering phases of the interview. Also, one should not pursue a specific line of inquiry longer than really necessary or to the exclusion of other unexplored areas. Excessive and highly detailed concentration on one area or line of inquiry will often convince the patient that there *must* be something there; otherwise the clinician would not be so intensely preoccupied with that area. In the same vein, rapid shifts in a line of inquiry may suggest to the patient that a given theme is not significant before it has been explored. Similarly, shifting from topic to topic and repeatedly returning to them can be confusing to the patient and reduce his accuracy of reporting. In brief, stay with a given line of inquiry as long as necessary to get all needed information, but no longer. Questions should always be framed for the specific patient being interviewed, taking into account his language skills, social and cultural background, and style of communication. With all patients, one should use simple, concise, non-technical language.

3   DEVELOPING A LINE OF INQUIRY

When the clinician decides to seek specific information, it is best obtained by gradually restricting the open-endedness of a series of questions presented to the patient. This is done by beginning with a most general and exploratory question pertinent to the body area or the topic in which the specific answer is sought. For example, in reviewing the respiratory system, if one wishes to find out whether the patient has pain in the upper right anterior area of the chest and whether it is made worse by respiration, an appropriate sequence of questions might be:

1. "How are your chest and lungs?"
2. (If symptoms are mentioned) "Could you please describe the discomfort (or pain)?"
3. "Where is the pain?" or "Could you please show me where the pain is?"
4. "Is the pain always the same or does it change?"
5. (If it changes) "What kind of things affect the pain?"
6. (If deep breathing is not mentioned) "Does deep breathing affect it at all?"

At any point in this sequence of questions, the patient might respond with all of the information, in his own words, that the physician is seeking. In fact, he might add a whole set of new and important associated data. If he has responded to the first question with all the needed information, the skilled interviewer asks no more to avoid the implication that he is interested primarily in pain or the effects of breathing. This encourages the patient to respond to other relatively open-ended questions with data that tend to be uninfluenced and unprejudiced by the clinician's inquiry.

If the patient responds in the negative to a relatively broad question, such as the first one listed above, the topic can be dropped at this point and the interviewer can move on to another area or topic of possible interest, particularly if the patient has demonstrated an easy responsiveness and the ability to communicate information effectively. If, however, the specific bit of information being sought, positive or negative, is of major importance in testing a given diagnostic possibility, it may be wise to pursue the line of questioning despite a negative response to the first one. One might go on to ask, "Do you have pain anywhere in the chest?" and even though this evokes a negative reply, ask, "Do you ever have discomfort in breathing?" While the wording of these questions encourages positive replies, this is the conservative approach in this circumstance. Finally, if the patient has denied symptoms and this is of crucial importance in establishing the diagnosis, it is justifiable to conclude with, "Then you are having no discomfort in your chest or lungs. Is that correct or have I misunderstood?" The exercise of clinical judgment is required in making the decision about how far to pursue specific information. It is based upon knowledge of the potential importance of the specific information being sought, as well as evaluation of the patient and his responses in the interview up to that point. Obviously, with a suggestible patient it is best not to pursue information to the extent described.

4   DIRECT QUESTIONING AFTER THE OPEN-ENDED PHASE OF THE INTERVIEW

Each symptom or bodily discomfort, whether reported by the patient spontaneously or elicited by the interviewer, requires specific qualifying information in order to be evaluated. It is usually best to delay inquiry into this qualifying information until after the patient's spontaneous account. Any necessary information that is not supplied by the patient should also be sought later, during the stage of the interview in which direct questions are being asked in order to fill in gaps. The qualifying information needed includes the following:

1. Location. Where is it experienced? If pain, does it radiate? If so, where? Under what circumstances does it do so?
2. Quality. What does it feel like? Is it dull or sharp, cutting, aching, throbbing, grinding? Other adjectives that may be used are "pressure," "crushing," "like a vise or band." If the discomfort is a limitation of function, as difficulty in breathing, a similar description of the character of the experience is needed.
3. Intensity. The terms the patient will use represent a mixture of subjective response to the pain as well as degree of severity. Though the description will range from mild to very severe or even unbearable, it should be evaluated in terms of the patient's personality or temperament. One man's severe pain is another's mild pain.
4. Quantitative aspects. How many? How often? How much? How big? Each of these may be applicable, depending on the type of discomfort or symptom reported.
5. Time of onset, duration, and frequency. If several symptoms are reported, what is their chronological relationship to each other, if any?
6. Setting. Under what circumstances does the symptom occur? Can it be related to the patient's location, his physical environment, or his social environment?
7. Aggravation and alleviation. Does anything make it worse or better?
8. Are there clearly related symptoms, limitations of function, or subjective responses, such as sensations of heat or cold, anxiety, depression, dizziness, faintness?
9. Has the patient taken medication or made other attempts to modify the symptoms chemically or physically?

Having reconstructed the patient's clinical problems and current symptoms, beginning with their onset, and having identified the course of the present illness, the interviewer should turn to the past medical history. Once again, the preferred approach is to begin with an open-ended inquiry. "How has your health been before this difficulty began?" is a good opening question. The usual response is a general one which requires elaboration. If the patient says something like "pretty good," or "fair," the interviewer should be facilitative. "Pretty good?" as a response will usually elicit qualifying data. If necessary, one can increase the specificity of questions until periods of ill health, as well as adequacy of general functioning during periods of good health, have been described. Ongoing problems, such as allergies, may call for a specific inquiry. For previous illnesses, the patient's report of a given diagnosis should not be accepted at face value. It is better to try to identify it from the account of onset, course, duration, type of treatment, and residual symptoms or functional limitation following the illness. This part of the interview will usually make it possible to place the present illness in the context of general health and previous adult illnesses and injuries.

The patient will usually not, however, give specific information about childhood health. If he does not, the interviewer begins again: "How was your health as a child?" Following the procedure of gradual increase in specificity of questions, one can inquire about specific illnesses, and finally, if need be, inquire about important childhood illnesses by name, as well as specific ones that might have a bearing on the present problem.

Other areas to be filled in with specific inquiries include the health status of the other family members and the relationships of the family members to each other and to the family as a unit.

If the patient's social history and the details of his current life situation with regard to family, work, life style, current emotional problems, and reactions to present stresses upon him have not emerged by this time, specific inquiries should now be directed to this area. A well-conducted interview will usually be characterized by the patient giving this information in context as he describes his present illness and past health.

5   DIRECT QUESTIONING TO DEVELOP NEW AREAS
OF INFORMATION

Direct questioning of patients is of two types. The first is that related to one or more of the problems the patient has already presented during the more open-ended phase of the interview, and the second is that designed to uncover other data or problems the patient has not remembered or has not described previously. Direct questioning about known problems should be carried out first and in order of the apparent relative importance of the problems. These questions should be designed to provide the clinician with a complete picture of these problems, in the light of his knowledge of the probable or possible disease processes involved. As always, the principle of asking the broadest questions first, followed by increasingly directed and specific questions, should be observed. This is a skill that can be attained only with practice. This requires a self-consciousness about one's phrasing of questions as a beginner. With experience, it becomes automatic.

Questions designed to elicit information the patient has not given voluntarily are commonly called the *Review of Systems* in the conventional medical record. This is usually taught as a list of fifty to one hundred questions covering cardinal disease manifestations of the body systems. In the name of thoroughness they are usually asked in checklist fashion of all patients as part of the so-called "complete work-up." No work-up can be truly complete, and much time is wasted by medical students and house officers in pursuit of this mythical ideal. It is our belief that if one tried instead for a better grasp of basic interviewing skills, the quality of the information available in medical records would be noticeably improved. Medical information can be obtained in checklist fashion more economically by a non-physician interviewer or health aide, by the use of a self-administered questionnaire, or by a computer-assisted data-gathering system. While useful to the physician, such data may be especially valuable for other medical purposes, such as health screening. It should not be a primary component of a physician's interview. Physicians should take advantage of their ability to do what cannot be done by fixed question lists: to listen to and interpret, in the light of one's knowledge of disease and of the patient, the uninfluenced story of a patient's problems as he sees them.

Nevertheless, it is useful to give the patient an opportunity to recall and describe complaints and observations not volunteered previously in the interview. The basic technique involved is the same as that already described for questioning the patient for amplification of information already obtained. A general, open-ended question, directed only enough to indicate the organ, system, area of the body, or function to which you wish the patient to attend, is asked first. If the patient replies negatively or gives only inconsequential information, the interviewer may move on. The next similar question is then posed. In certain areas, and with certain patients, second and third more specific questions may be asked. For example, in questioning a patient about possible cardiac dysfunction or disease, the first question might be, "Have you ever had any problems with your heart, or not?" If the reply is "no" it might be appropriate to ask a fifty-year-old obese male, "Do you have any shortness of breath when you are exerting yourself?" and "Do you have any pain in your chest brought on by hard work or exercise?" Additional specific questions may be asked based upon the level of suspicion created by other aspects of the situation. These would include the circumstances in which the patient is seen, his appearance, and what he has said earlier in the interview. A rote list of perfunctory questions should be avoided at all costs. On the other hand, each clinician tends to develop his own system-directed inquiries which he can use when needed.

What is usually termed the system review is best thought of as an organizing device and an aid to the memory. That is, after obtaining an account of the present illness and the past health history as an adult and child, and after filling in significant gaps through direct inquiry, it is well to consider whether all organ systems and areas of the body that could be of relevance to the assessment of the present state of health or illness have been covered. Inquiries can then be made, if indicated, either during the physical examination or just prior to undertaking it. The same systematic order of conducting the physical examination supplies the major headings for this phase of data collection. A well-conducted interview will usually have brought out most of the information. The remainder is easily obtained just prior to examining each system or area.

6 OBTAINING INFORMATION ABOUT SEXUALITY

The sexual history is an integral part of the initial diagnostic interview. Many physical and emotional problems can cause sexual dysfunction, as can some medications. Sexual preferences and practices can place certain patients at risk for specific illnesses. Sexual concerns and problems may underly somatic complaints.

It is the rare patient who spontaneously volunteers specific sexual information, so it is usually the clinician who has to take the initiative through direct questioning. Many clinicians find it very difficult to ask their patients about sexual matters. This mutual discomfort can lead to an inadequate evaluation of the patient's sexuality, or to no evaluation at all.

When to obtain the sexual history depends on the nature of the patient's problems and his willingness to report them. If the patient has come for help with a sexual problems, such as impotence, the sexual history should be explored early in the interview. If the patient exhibits symptoms of a condition associated with certain sexual practices, such as hepatitis B, if he has an illness that can cause sexual dysfunction, such as diabetes, or if he is taking a medication that can cause sexual problems, the sexual history should be obtained during the evaluation of that complaint. If the patient's problem is clearly unrelated to his sexuality, the sexual history can wait until late in the interview. This permits greater rapport and trust to be established before beginning a discussion of this sensitive topic.

It is an error to assume that any patient, be he six or ninety-six, single or married, is not sexually active or has no sexual concerns.

However, it is also unnecessary to obtain an exhaustive sexual history from every patient. The clinician needs to obtain enough information to adequately assess the patient's physical and emotional health, no more and no less. To accomplish this, five areas should be explored:

1. What is the patient's sexual *preference?* (e.g., heterosexual, homosexual, or bisexual)
2. What are the patient's sexual *practices?* (e.g., vaginal, oral, or anal intercourse; masturbation, fetishism)
3. Is the patient *satisfied* with his current sexual relationship(s)?
4. Does the patient have any sexual *problems* or *concerns?*
5. Does the patient have any *questions* about sexuality?

It requires a special effort not to introduce bias when interviewing patients about their sexuality. If the patient perceives that the clinician disapproves of anything the patient has said about his sexuality, he may withhold important information. The clinician may communicate disapproval through an unfortunate choice of words, by not asking certain questions, or by a facial expression. While there are techniques to minimize the introduction of bias, every clinician also must become familiar with the various expressions of human sexuality if he is to be comfortable talking with patients whose preferences and practices differ from his own.

If the patient has not initiated a discussion of his sexuality, it falls to the clinician to do so. The best way to proceed is to say something like, "As you know, I am responsible for helping you maintain your health in all areas. To do this, it may be helpful if I know about your sexual adjustment and any concerns you might have. Many people are uncomfortable talking about sex. How do you feel about discussing it?" This approach places the sexual history under the broader issue of the patient's well-being, while offering the patient both reassurance and support.

Once the interviewer is fairly certain that any anxiety the patient has is tolerable enough for him to talk about sex, the interviewer should proceed with more directive questioning. Questions should be phrased in ways that avoid making any assumptions about the number and gender of the patient's sexual partner(s). A question like "Are you currently sexually active?" makes no assumptions at all, but it is specific enough to begin a discussion.

It is also a good idea to use the words "partner" or "partners" until the number and gender(s) of the patient's sexual companions are known, even if the patient is married and therefore likely to be heterosexual and monogamous. As with all interviewing, the clinician must avoid using language that is too technical. The best approach is to use the sexual terms that the patient uses, but in doing so it is important that the clinician be sure that he and the patient both understand what the term means. Another technique that can be helpful is the "ubiquity" question, one that assumes that most people have experienced the subject under discussion.[4] Examples of ubiquity questions include: "When did you *first* experience . . ." or "*When* or *how* did you first learn about . . ." rather than "Have you *ever* experienced . . ." or "*Do* you know about . . ."

Finally, it is always best to proceed from less sensitive to more sensitive subjects during the interview. The more rapport between clinician and patient, the more willing the patient will be to discuss any unusual or deviant sexual practices. At the end of the sexual history, it is a good idea to close with a statement that leaves the area open to future discussion.

There is one group of patients with whom the sexual history can generally be omitted: children. However, the clinician should always keep in mind the fact that there are children who are involved in sexual activities. If there is evidence that this is the case, it is vital that a sexual history be obtained. While specific techniques for interviewing children are discussed in Chapter 6, we offer the following guidelines on talking to children about sexuality:

1. Children who are victims of incest or other sexual molestation have often been threatened with harm should they ever "tell anyone." They need to be approached gently, and a high degree of trust must be established before asking specific questions.

2. Unless it is the parents who suspect that the child has been involved in sexual activities and raise the question, the interview should not take place in the parents' presence.
3. Once trust has been established, the best way to approach the subject of sexuality is to talk about touching. While many children know sexual words, most also know that they're not supposed to say them, so the use of such words is counterproductive. Instead, if the clinician helps the child identify how he likes to be touched (good-night kisses, hugs, and so forth), then the clinician can ask the child about other kinds of touching and whether or not he's ever been touched in a way he didn't understand, didn't like, or didn't want.

The importance of making an effort to obtain a sexual history from a child when sexual abuse is suspected cannot be stressed enough. In the vast majority of cases, children never tell their parents what has happened, either because of fear or shame. Their only possible source of help and protection are the other trusted adult authority figures in their lives, most often teachers or clinicians.

7   THE MENTAL STATUS EXAMINATION

Assessment of mental status occurs whenever the clinician and the patient are together. No clinical examination is complete without this assessment. In many, if not most, instances very few specific inquiries need be made since it can be easily ascertained whether or not the areas of mental functioning with which the examiner is concerned are within normal limits. This means, however, that the examiner has had these areas of mental functioning in mind throughout the interview. While the patient tells his story, the interviewer concerns himself with both content and process. He listens to what the patient says and to how he says it. If he then gets evidence that the patient's mental status needs closer scrutiny, he can make the necessary inquiries. In the case of some patients, particularly children and those who are defensive, it may be neces-

sary to interview other family members in order to complete the
examination.

The areas to be examined in a thorough mental status examination include appearance and behavior, speech, mood, thought
content, and orientation and cognition.

Appearance and Behavior

As the patient enters the room, the examiner notes his posture or
carriage, dress, facial expression, and attitude. The depressed patient, for example, will usually look sad or washed-out, move slowly,
and appear to be hesitant or unsure. When seated, his shoulders
will droop and his facial expression will be characterized by a
downturned mouth and a bleak or unhappy look. On the other
hand, the anxious patient will transmit a look of apprehension,
will often be restless or even tremulous, and may perspire freely.
One should note the patient's dress, the feeling tone transmitted
by his facial expression (anger, bewilderment, fear, blandness, sadness, and so forth), his attitude toward the interviewer, and the
interviewer's response.

Speech

How the patient talks will give important diagnostic clues. Tone
of voice, inflection, volume (very loud or very soft), continuity
(Does the patient speak rapidly, slowly, or haltingly? Are there
long periods of silence?), and organization (coherence, logicality,
ability to give an account without rambling into unrelated irrele-
vancies or excessive detail) are the important features to note.

Mood

How does the patient feel? If he does not tell you spontaneously,
an inquiry is in order. A confrontation about observed evidence of
a disturbance in mood is the preferred approach when possible.
Some patients are aware of feeling depressed or anxious or of having disturbing fluctuations of mood and freely volunteer this information. Others will not speak about it until they are asked or

confronted with your observations about their mood. And there are patients who have disturbances of mood but deny this, as though it might just "go away" if they pretend it's not there. For this reason the interviewer should check his own impression of the patient's mood against the patient's description. Hints about suicidal tendencies should be followed up and thoroughly explored. Other disturbances of mood that may be reported are feelings of unreality or of detachment. Some patients will say, "I don't feel anything," a very distressing state akin to severe and chronic depression.

Thought Content

What are the patient's preoccupations and how realistic do they appear to be? Does he feel that he is in control of his thoughts? If not, what sort of loss of control is he experiencing? For example, some people experience obsessions—repetitive, often unpleasant, uncontrollable thoughts that they find intrusive and upsetting. Others experience delusions—for example, they insist that their minds are being controlled by some outside force—and these delusions may not be unpleasant at all. Still others experience hallucinations, such as hearing voices, and they are sometimes preoccupied with these internal dialogues to the point of intermittently responding to the voices rather than to the interviewer.

Orientation and Cognition

In the usual diagnostic interview with a general medical patient this is not a detailed examination. But if it becomes apparent that the patient has serious neuropsychiatric problems, the examination of the patient's cognitive function should be carried out in some detail. The reliability of the patient's history and his ability to understand the nature of his problem and to participate in his treatment depend upon his being able to learn and remember. If these functions are in some way compromised, family members or other caretakers will have to be called upon to supply the patient's history and to be actively involved in his care.

Cognitive testing consists of asking a series of formal questions borrowed from diagnostic psychological tests. These are described in standard textbooks of psychiatry. In the non-psychiatric patient, it is necessary to note only whether the patient is oriented (that is, aware of who he is, where he is, the date, and time), has the ability to pay attention to what is happening, and is capable of ordinary concentration. One should also note defects of memory, ability to do abstract reasoning, evidence of reasonably good or of poor judgment, and adequacy of perception—visual, auditory, and tactile.

While it is very likely that defects of perception and orientation will become apparent in the course of a well-conducted interview, one can be misled by patients who have brain damage and who confabulate. Such patients will fill in the gaps in their defective memory with facts and details manufactured on the spot. If these are not blatantly self-contradictory, the examiner may not recognize them as confabulations. If the interviewer has any clue that brain damage, such as from chronic alcoholism, is part of the problem, it is well to inquire directly about the date, time, and place. Such a patient commonly will not be able to state the day, month, and year; nor will he be able to account satisfactorily for recent periods of time.

8   INTERVIEWING DURING THE PHYSICAL EXAMINATION

Communication with the patient should not be allowed to lapse during performance of the physical examination. Silence on the part of the physician as he examines may be regarded as ominous by the apprehensive patient. If the patient feels that silence is expected by the physician, he may not respond if, as a result of some maneuver of the physical examination, he recalls a fact he would like to add to the information already given. The physical examination should be orderly and comprehensive, requirements best satisfied by employing an unvarying, basic routine. The inexperienced physician may find it difficult to divide his attention between what he is doing and observing and what the patient is saying that might be of importance. However, the examiner should learn to continue speaking with the patient while examining him, if for no other reason than to relieve tension and maintain open lines of communication with the patient. This is still another reason for using the time of the physical examination to complete the organ- and system-directed inquiry, previously described as the Review of Systems. It is most appropriate to do it at this time because the inquiry and the physical examination, properly performed, mutually reinforce each other. The questions with the related examination procedure strongly stimulate recall by the patient. The patient's responses help to direct the physician's examining procedure and his interpretations of what he observes. Time is also saved. If the physician does question the patient as he examines him, he should of course use the technique we have emphasized of first asking the most open-ended question pertinent to the area under investigation, followed by increasingly specific questions as necessary. Timing of the questions is crucial; the first question should always be posed *before* beginning to examine a given area. The patient will then respond while the area is being examined, unless silence is needed to permit auscultation. In that case, permit the patient to answer before asking him for the period of silence needed while you listen. If the first question about a given organ or system is asked during or after examining it, the patient may take this to mean that a significant abnormality has been encountered. This creates anxiety and the patient is then likely to be more interested in finding out what you have discovered than in providing information. While it is difficult to learn to maintain the proper timing relationship of questioning and examining, with questions just leading the related examination procedure, it is a most useful skill that can be acquired by experience if it is regularly practiced.

9 EXAMINING THE ANXIOUS PATIENT

If a patient is becoming visibly anxious during the physical examination, in spite of the precautions noted, it is appropriate to give reassurance periodically with casual comments on the normality of certain of the findings. If a patient's level of anxiety is rising, it almost always inhibits his communication. If you find that open-ended questions yield progressively less information from the patient and more and more highly specific questions are required, it is reasonable to assume that the patient is becoming increasingly anxious. It is well to interrupt the examination at this point and inquire into this. The line of questioning may have been too highly directive. The patient may be becoming anxious or depressed. Something may have suggested to the patient that you are not really interested in him or are not to be trusted. Or you may have unwittingly provoked anxiety by a variety of unintentional errors of omission or commission. For example, when a patient is alone and unclothed in an austere examining room and has a prolonged wait for the doctor, he will very likely become anxious and depressed or angry. It is always important to examine such a situation critically. The preferred approach is to confront the patient supportively with your observations about his communication and manner. Very often, then, he will tell you what is creating the inhibition. Often, too, some information or reassurance can be given that will put the patient much more at ease. Interviewing the anxious patient is discussed in Chapter 4.

10   INTERVIEWING PATIENTS WITH COMMUNICATION DIFFICULTIES

Special problems are encountered in interviewing patients who are deaf, blind, aphonic, aphasic, or unable to speak a language in which the interviewer is fluent. The delirious patient might be added to this list also. Although each of these situations is different, there are certain general principles in interviewing common to them all. These derive from the fundamental principles of open-ended interviewing. Remember that the purpose of an interview is to gather pertinent information on which a medical intervention may be based and to create a relationship with the patient.

Developing a relationship with patients with whom communication is difficult may be even more important than doing so with the fully communicative patient. Many people with communication handicaps live in relative isolation. They form friendships slowly and with difficulty. Some are suspicious, feeling a need for constant vigilance because of difficulty in perceiving what is going on around them. The development of a relationship in these circumstances must be pursued deliberately and with sensitivity, with special emphasis on the non-verbal communication one ordinarily uses unconsciously. A well-timed reaching out to touch the patient by a handshake, smile, or gesture may communicate more than words. People with such handicaps are commonly highly attuned to insincerity. It is better to move slowly and preserve genuineness, responding to your own feelings, than to attempt to force a friendly relationship for which neither you nor the patient is ready.

Except for certain aphasic patients with obvious extensive brain damage, or severely delirious patients, it is important to assess the communication-impaired patient's intellect. It is very likely to be entirely intact. Communication deficits may give an impression of reduced mental or cognitive function. Accordingly, the interviewer may respond inappropriately and to bad effect by oversimplifying his normal mode of speaking or by dealing with an adult patient in a child-like way. This can have deleterious effects on the ultimate development of an effective clinician-patient relationship.

It is also valuable to record details of the best way to communicate with these patients in their medical records, including names and addresses of communicators, for future use and for use by other people.

The Use of Communicators

At times it may be necessary to employ an intermediary in interviewing patients with communication problems. This may be a person able to use sign language, a translator, or a family member who understands the speech of a dysarthric patient. Under these circumstances, the relationship with the patient can become confused, since it is easy to develop a relationship with the intermediary and not with the patient. It is important, then, to focus first on the patient and secondarily on the communication. If the communicator has a relationship of significance with the patient, this should be taken into account. It is generally helpful to look at the patient, both when posing inquiries to be translated and while listening to replies. At times, as the reply is being given, the patient will add significant non-verbal cues to which the interviewer can respond. In general, the patient should be present during all communications with the third person. Confidentiality must be maintained by the communicator and the patient must be assured of this, particularly when they are not acquainted. If sensitive matters are discussed, it is best to employ a third person not known to the patient when possible. The patient may find it difficult or impossible to discuss such matters with an acquaintance or family member.

Interviewing the Deaf and Hearing-Impaired Patient

Hearing impairment occurs most commonly with older patients, but it may occur with patients of any age group. It can pose great difficulty to the interview. If the patient has some residual hearing, first find out how to use it to the best advantage. Usually the patient will tell you how to proceed if asked directly at the outset. Patients who have hearing aids should be encouraged to use them, even though they may not be wearing them at the moment. It may be wise to defer the interview until the hearing aid is available.

If the patient is able to lip-read and has adequate phonation, useful communication can usually be established. Sit in a location where you are easily seen, in a well-lighted room, and face the patient when speaking. Articulate normally; do not over-articulate, as this may be more difficult for the patient to interpret than normal speech. Speak at a moderate, even pace. Words not understood can be spelled orally or written. Patients vary widely in this skill. At times it is only marginally useful, and another mode of communication may be more satisfactory to both interviewer and patient.

Interviewing the Mute or Aphonic Patient

If the patient knows sign language, use of a communicator skilled in it is usually preferable, as the process is interactive, faster, and more comfortable for the patient. Writing can supplement signing, but it is slow, may be difficult for people who are ill or have additional physical handicaps, and should be avoided when possible. If necessary, we prefer to carry out written communications with patients by employing a writing pad and a soft pencil rather than an erasable slate, which some patients carry for other brief communications. Paper and pencil provide a record from which to work later. At times it is useful to ask the patient to write out the history of the illness as a preliminary to a more interactive interview. This conforms to good interviewing practice in that such a document is open-ended in structure and is relatively uninfluenced by the interviewer. Written communication, of course, depends substantially on the extent of the patient's literacy. Neglected deaf and mute patients may not be able to express themselves well in written communication. Similarly, small degrees of depressed brain function inhibit written communication more than would be experienced in the ordinary verbal code. Thus, there are many circumstances when supplementary data from an informant, as discussed in Chapter 6, is necessary. If the communication problem is severe, it may be appropriate to interview informants prior to interviewing the patient so that the limited communication possible with the patient is focused on the most important issues that need to be resolved prior to therapy.

Interviewing Blind Patients

We tend to underestimate the limitations on communication imposed by blindness because we can talk with the blind freely. Many blind people are particularly articulate conversationalists. We fail to recognize that the whole range of visual, non-verbal cues of the interview are denied the blind patient. Instead, the blind person employs a highly developed compensation in interpreting a whole range of sounds to supplement the verbal exchange. From there he determines the mood, character, style, and attitudes of the interviewer. Tone of voice, the sounds of significant body movements, clearing the throat, laughter, and a host of other cues of which sighted persons are only marginally aware are the data blind persons detect and interpret with great acuity. These non-visual cues may or may not reflect a picture congruent with one that a sighted person would receive in a similar interview. There is thus a smaller and more fragile margin for misunderstanding as the relationship of the patient and interviewer develops.

Blind people may want to be told something of the surroundings into which they are taken (for example, an examining room or office); inform the patient of the approximate size and shape of the room, where the major items of furniture are located, and the locations of entrances, curtains, and the like. All other people present, if any, and their locations should be identified at the outset in nearly every circumstance. The other people present may say a few words to establish their voice pattern for the patient. If you move from one part of the room to another, describe what you are doing. This should be done in a matter-of-fact, brief way. The patient should be given an opportunity to ask questions about the environment before the interview begins.

Blind people vary a great deal in the amount of help they need or want in moving around, finding things, and tending to everyday needs. Do not preempt their decisions; rather, ask if your help is needed when you feel it may be. Older, otherwise infirm people and those recently blind will need more assistance than those who have been blind for a long time and who have received special training in daily living activities. Gently lead—do not push—a blind person whom you are helping to move. The objective should be to keep intact the patient's sense of self-sufficiency, which may have been hard-won, just as in the case of the physically handicapped.

Above all, avoid raising the level of your ordinary conversational tone of voice, changing the normal pace of your speech, overarticulating, or speaking in short, simplified sentences. Surprisingly, blind people are often thoughtlessly dealt with in this way. They find it highly offensive, a gross manifestation of insensitivity, or at best ridiculous. The effect of this error on the potential doctor-patient relationship needs no comment.

In summary, patients with handicaps in communication present special problems in interviewing that commonly can be overcome by relatively simple means properly employed. The basic principles of interviewing still apply in these circumstances. Sensitivity of the interviewer to the individual patient and his special circumstances is paramount. The importance of a good, workable, therapeutic relationship between interviewer and patient must not be neglected by focusing communication strictly on the collection of data.

REFERENCES

1. These introductory paragraphs are a distillation of portions of Chapter 2, "The Nature of Medical Information and the Social Context of the Interview," from the second edition of *Interviewing and Patient Care*.
2. Payne, S. L., *The Art of Asking Questions*. Princeton, N.J.: Princeton University Press, 1951.
3. Leigh, Hoyle, and Morton F. Reiser, *The Patient: Biological, Psychological, and Social Dimensions of Medical Practice*. New York: Plenum Medical Book Company, 1980.
4. Green, R., *Human Sexuality: A Health Practitioner's Text*, Second Edition. Baltimore, MD., Williams & Wilkins, 1979. Page 25.

4

EMOTIONAL AND BEHAVIORAL RESPONSES TO ILLNESS AND TO THE INTERVIEWER

1 PSYCHOLOGICAL REACTIONS TO ILLNESS

Blum[1] describes ten major reactions, one or more of which is likely to characterize a patient's response to becoming sick. They are: depression and self-rejection; fear; counterphobia; anxiety; frustration and anger; withdrawal or apathy; exaggeration of symptoms; regression; dependency; and self-centeredness. These general emotional reactions are not specific to any particular illness and are separate from the physiologic effects of any particular disease. They are, however, characteristic of that individual's usual response to stress or to anxiety-provoking situations. Later in this chapter we will discuss some ways of dealing with these responses during the interview.

Psychological reactions to illness begin before the individual defines himself as sick and before he seeks help. Lederer[2] suggested that the responses of the sick to their illness could be described in three phases: first, the transition period from health to illness; second, the period of "accepted" illness; and third, convalescence. In the transition period from health to illness, Lederer pointed out, most persons first become aware of some undesirable, unpleasant, and painful sensations, as well as a reduction in strength and stam-

and to communicate to others that he is not afraid. The idea that illness could result in being helpless is so intolerable that behavior designed to demonstrate the opposite is acted out.

A forty-two-year-old businessman succeeded in building a large and diversified company largely through his own efforts. He was accustomed to being involved in a number of business deals at any given time and kept constantly in touch with all his operations, even having a telephone in his automobile. When admitted to the hospital for examination, though seriously ill and in great discomfort, he was unable to lie in bed. He walked around the room, made business phone calls, and repeatedly interrupted the student who was attempting to conduct an initial diagnostic interview.

The usual indication that a patient is becoming very anxious is an intensification of his customary ways of coping with the world. For instance, the compulsive patient who has a need to be organized and to keep the world orderly and predictable will, on falling ill, become much more compulsive and extremely "fussy." He will insist on even more orderliness, predictability and neatness, or cleanliness than usual.

A twenty-two-year-old college student was admitted to the hospital for examination because of weakness, diarrhea, weight loss, abdominal pain, and evidence of anemia. He was a highly organized, orderly, and neat individual who was described as "compulsive." In the hospital, he complained of failure to collect his stool specimens and lack of punctuality with schedules, even though neither complaint was warranted. He became upset if he did not receive a new hospital gown each day, even though his was not dirty.

The anxious patient may be difficult to interview until the anxiety itself has been discussed. The patient who fears helplessness reacts best when the clinician's air of competence and concern indicates that he can be trusted; when he feels that he is receiving full and complete explanations in answer to his questions, reducing the ambiguity of the situation; and when efforts are made to reduce his sense of helplessness by allowing him to be as active as the situation permits.

Dependency. The social role of patient means that passivity and reliance on others or, in other words, dependency is expected. In the reasonably flexible individual, being dependent when one has become a patient does not pose difficulties. It is possible for individuals who are ordinarily quite independent to accept dependence on the physician, nurses, and medical staff when they become patients. But there are individuals whose need to be independent and active is very strong and who have kept up a constant battle to ward off any impulse to be dependent. For them, to be cared for is quite unacceptable. Becoming a patient represents a temptation to them that is very threatening. These are the patients who are most likely to have a counterphobic response to their anxiety. They may put off going to the doctor or clinic, and once there they may minimize their symptoms for fear of being ordered to bed.

Inability to Accept Warmth or Tenderness. Blum has pointed out that popular writing in psychology emphasizes the shame which can attend anger and sexual desires but that reluctance to experience tenderness is rarely mentioned. Tenderness refers to sympathetic and affectionate acts by which a person expresses love and concern for another person. Much of the care patients receive from family, friends, and medical personnel is tender care. This makes some people anxious.

Such patients when interviewed, particularly if they are seriously ill and in a hospital bed, become brusque and gruff and speak in distant or irritable tones. Their behavior communicates "keep your distance" and can be upsetting to an interviewer who is trying to be friendly and helpful. It may be necessary for the interviewer to examine his own behavior. To be overly solicitous or warm may be far too threatening to the patient. An increase in the interviewer's own reserve may reduce the discomfort of such a patient.

Fear of Expressing Anger. There are many things that can provoke anger in a patient. A patient who arrives on time for a two o'clock appointment and then has a forty-five-minute wait in the reception room before the interview begins has a legitimate source of anger, for example. Anger can be an appropriate response to many of the circumstances of being a hospital patient. Inattentive personnel and failure to respond to the patient's needs are common, though not always intentional, occurrences in the hospital. But the situation of being helpless and dependent on others makes a patient especially sensitive to failure to meet his needs. Anger is a common response.

However, there are people who cannot permit themselves to express anger. With such a patient, anxiety over helplessness together with a fear of upsetting those on whom he must depend, potentiates his fear of expressing anger and increases his anxiety. This is often reinforced by physicians and nurses whose behavior communicates to the patient that they will not accept his anger and may retaliate. Yet, an important dimension of the clinician's role is to encourage expressions of such anger and to tolerate it even when it seems somewhat unreasonable. Only then can the patient's anxiety over his anger be reduced.

Depression

Schwab *et al.* studied the medical records of patients referred for consultation at the University of Florida Teaching Hospital and found that the term *"depressed"* could be found in 32 per cent of all the records they studied.[5] It is probable, however, that depression accompanies every severe illness. Research on responses of children to separation from their mothers, on bereavement, and on psychosomatic illness[6,7,8] all lend strong support to the view that depression is a psycho-physiologic response to loss, including loss of self-esteem. Thus, while depression may be the underlying problem in a large proportion of those patients who consult their physician with complaints of fatigue, weakness, lack of energy, insomnia, backache, or headache, depression as a response to illness is equally common, if not more so. Characteristically, depressed people have feelings of worthlessness, hopelessness, apathy, and guilt, together with a profoundly empty or lonely feeling. The depression will be manifested in the patient's manner, tone of voice, posture, and speech. Thinking is slow, speech is sparse, and voice volume is low. Hopelessness and sadness are reflected in the patient's drooping shoulders, downturned mouth, and lackluster eyes. A severely depressed patient will volunteer little and will respond to questions with brief, relatively uninformative answers. This will reduce the amount of information that can be obtained about the onset and development of the illness. Many of these patients are people for whom having an illness is equivalent to being useless or "bad." Self-accusation may also be a component in depressive response to illness in instances where a patient believes he has not taken proper care of himself or has ignored advice given to him previously by his physician. Mild to moderate depression can be dealt with relatively easily during the interview, and good interviewing technique may bring some relief of the depressive symptoms. Severe depression can, however, be a major complication of the illness as well as of the interview itself.

Depressive reactions to illness may be characterized by apathetic withdrawal with silences. In such an instance a confrontation can be very helpful. A statement like "You look very sad" or "You look depressed" gives the patient the opportunity to talk about his depressed feelings. It is usually necessary to be more active in interviewing a depressed patient than one would be with other types of patients. More direct questions have to be asked and these are usually asked earlier in the interview than with a patient who is more communicative.

A special problem may be posed by the patient who begins to cry during an interview. Many clinicians find this uncomfortable. However, it may be of considerable help both to the patient and to the interviewer. Fighting tears often results in the patient not being able to speak. Weeping, on the other hand, often affords relief of severe depressive feelings and may make it possible for the patient to resume his account. It may also help the patient to feel closer to the clinician. The appropriate response of the interviewer is to maintain a sympathetic silence while the patient cries and respond with a supportive remark thereafter (e.g., "You must be feeling very bad"). A common error, usually stemming from the

interviewer's discomfort, is to interrupt the crying with reassuring
or supportive remarks before the patient has had a chance to "cry
it out." It is better to wait patiently, to provide a tissue if necessary, to respond with sympathetic support after the patient has
stopped crying, and to make no effort to resume the interview
until then.

When a patient is on the verge of tears and this is clearly making it difficult for him to speak, it is often helpful to invite the crying with a confrontation: "You look like you are about to cry."
The opportunity to cry, followed by the support offered by the
clinician, will permit the interview to continue—and it can be
therapeutic.

Denial

There are some patients whose customary way of dealing with
frightening ideas or impulses is by never permitting them to enter
their minds. On becoming ill, such patients must deny to themselves that such a thing has happened or that they need treatment.
Consequently, they minimize or completely deny symptoms and
consciously or unconsciously mislead the interviewer. Such patients
are never completely aware of the degree to which they withhold,
modify, or alter significant information. Other patients who are
not ordinarily deniers will consciously withhold or distort information because they are ashamed or fearful of the consequences of
revealing it. Morgan and Engel[9] point out that denial or withhold-
ing is usually betrayed by the obvious disparity between the patient's condition and how he reports it. He may overstate how well
he feels or be overly vehement about the non-existence of a symptom. A tendency to dismiss all symptoms with such words as
"only" or "a little" should cue the interviewer to the fact that the
patient is using denial. Those patients who consciously withhold
information often respond with evidence of discomfort or embarrassment which reveal that a sensitive topic is under discussion
about which the patient would rather not say too much.

Patients who always deal with unacceptable thoughts and feelings by denying them are not reliable informants about their own

illnesses. If the interviewer clarifies his role at the outset and can create confidence in himself, he may be able to reduce the amount of denial used by the patient. But, as Morgan and Engel point out, with this type of patient it is essential to interview a reliable informant as well. They warn, however, that in almost all instances the patient should not be confronted with the information obtained from the outside source.[10]

In subsequent interviews, with the development of a good clinician-patient relationship, the degree of denial used by the patient may be reduced markedly or, in the case of the conscious withholder, disappear completely.

Projection

There are individuals who deal with all perceived internal dangers through projection. They control fear by shifting it from mysterious and potentially dangerous internal events to more concrete, more understandable, and potentially more controllable targets outside themselves, which they misperceive as the source of the danger. Like denial, projection is usually a character trait, though it may be relatively undetectable until the individual begins to become aware that he is feeling ill. Such patients respond to the discomfort and limitation of function that are part of the transition from health to illness by becoming suspicious of everyone around them, including the physician and other health professionals they encounter in seeking help. These patients tend to be distrustful as a matter of course but can tolerate their distrust during communication under ordinary circumstances. However, the internal danger to continued existence that they perceive in illness exacerbates their distrust since much more than usual is now at stake. Interviewing such patients is a difficult task at best. During the interview, the patient may angrily burst out with "Why do you want to know that?" The most insignificant action may be construed by the patient to mean that the interviewer is not to be trusted and can create anger or accusations of bad faith or will. The interviewer or anyone who is trying to be helpful may be bewildered and annoyed by such attacks. When a patient becomes clearly suspicious and angry at the introduction of a topic into the interview, the interviewer would be well advised to back off for the moment. The best attitude toward paranoid patients is tactful firmness, avoidance of angry responses to the patient, consistency, and patience. Only in time and with consistency will it be possible to build a sense of trust in the patient, if at all. If all the desired information cannot be obtained in one interview, the clinician must be patient and use as many interviews as necessary to collect the needed data. With the paranoid patient, it is a good idea not to interview collateral sources except with the permission of the patient and in his presence.

2   RESPONSES TO THE DOCTOR

The doctor-patient relationship tends to bring out attitudes and behavior reflecting previous relationships with other authorities or skilled technicians whose competence had an important bearing on the individual's comfort or welfare.[11] This is also true of the nurse and the social worker, but probably to a somewhat lesser degree. The more the patient feels that he is sick, and to that extent more helpless and dependent, the more likely it is that his attitude toward the doctor will reflect a great deal of these previously learned attitudes. These attitudes are often manifested in ways that appear totally irrational to the interviewer. A patient who has had an angry, competitive relationship with his father, perceiving the physician as a powerful authority, may become antagonistic, sarcastic, and competitive even though the doctor has done nothing that would ordinarily elicit such a response. Female clinicians often encounter irrational responses based on the patient's early experiences with being mothered.

There is also the likelihood of an irrational response to the doctor, nurse, or other clinician as succorer or sympathy giver. Because the patient is usually in pain, is anxious, and is aware of a threat, possibly of death or at least of impaired function, his need for attention and sympathy is far greater than it is at other times. He is therefore very likely to respond in ways that reflect his relationship with his mother or other individuals to whom he turned for love and sympathy for his childhood discomforts. If these were satisfying experiences, he may be a relaxed and appropriately compliant patient. If they were frustrating experiences, he may approach the clinician with a mixture of fear, suspicion, and expectation of disappointment. If, as is so often the case with individuals who had chronic illness in childhood, the patient obtained attention and sympathy mostly through illness, he may embrace the role of patient and exploit it for as much sympathetic attention as he can get.

Still another determinant of the patient's response to the clinician is the experiences he has had in the past in getting health care. For some people, particularly those raised in urban ghettos who obtained health care in clinics at large public hospitals, the matter of going to the doctor evokes memories of long waits, impersonal and dehumanizing encounters, and disregard for privacy. Chronic illness in childhood requiring painful procedures may make every visit to the doctor a dreaded event.

In other words, the interaction between doctor and patient, as well as between nurse and patient or other health professionals to whom the patient turns for help when sick, is highly charged with emotion. This will significantly affect the patient's interview behavior. Some of the more common responses that can pose problems for the interviewer include silence, over-talkativeness, seductiveness, anger, aggressively demanding behavior, suspicion and distrust, and passive or dependent behavior.

The Silent Patient

With most patients, occasional silences are not uncommon during an interview. Silences of up to half a minute (which may feel quite protracted, even interminable, to the interviewer) usually mean that the patient is trying to recall something or is silently debating to himself whether to speak about a given topic or not. This is discussed at length in Chapter 3. Many interviewers, and most beginners, do not tolerate such silences well and some interviewers never permit a patient the luxury of a period of silence.

This may reflect, in part, the clinician's lack of comfort with the doctor-patient relationship since silences are not uncommon in conversations with people with whom one has a reasonably close social relationship. It may also partly reflect the clinician's feeling that he has a task to perform, to be carried out with maximum efficiency and dispatch. The most common reason clinicians interrupt silences is their own tension. Most interviewers tend to over-estimate the duration of a silence. A useful exercise is to experiment with estimating the length of timed silences during interviews before actually checking the time. With practice one can learn to permit silence until the patient's tension suggests a confrontation or until the patient speaks.

> The patient has been talking about her low back pain. The backache began during her first pregnancy, became worse after her second pregnancy, and is now constant. There is a note of marked discontent in her voice. After a few minutes she falls silent.
>
> *(After about 20 seconds)*
> INTERVIEWER: Anything else?
> *(Silence—20 seconds. The patient looks more depressed.)*
> INTERVIEWER: You look quite unhappy.
> *(Silence—15 seconds)*
> PATIENT: I feel just awful. The children are just too much for me. All that lifting and carrying hurts my back so much. And I get no help from Jack. *(Tears appear.)* Oh, I just knew if I talked about it, I'd start to cry.

There are patients, however, who remain silent for long periods of time, or fall silent frequently. The interviewer may have the feeling that he is constantly pushing the patient to keep communication going and obtain some information. This usually means that the patient is seriously depressed, which may be part of the illness or a response to it. Questioning about symptoms of depression, as well as careful observation for the classic signs of depression in the patient's facial expression, posture, and attitude, will clarify the diagnosis. Prolonged and repeated silences may also be a manifestation of an organic brain disease or a psychosis.

There are instances when prolonged or repeated silences result from poor interviewing technique. Clumsy or insensitive handling of the opening phase of the interview, too many specific questions asked too early in the interview, too many interruptions, or tactless remarks may result in silences and brief answers which reflect withdrawal and, usually, an offended patient.

The Over-talkative Patient

A most difficult problem for beginner and experienced interviewer alike is the over-talkative patient. This patient may be seen as a barrier to getting a day's work done with reasonable efficiency. He very often frustrates the clinician's efforts to get sufficient relevant information within reasonable time limits, and he is usually a major source of irritation to him. Such a patient, then, slows down the clinician and imposes a burden of self-restraint upon him. This is not, however, the only reason that such patients are irritating to the interviewer. There is usually an aggressive quality to such a patient's communication which has a controlling or dominating effect. One type of over-talkative patient is the obsessional individual who insists on giving an over-detailed account, omitting nothing, not even the most trivial detail. In interviewing such a patient, one must be careful to avoid over-facilitating through encouraging nods, gestures, and phrases. Relatively specific questions should be introduced earlier in the sequence of the interview than might be done with a less obsessive patient. The interviewer should limit his show of interest when the patient is supplying a great deal of trivial detail but show greater interest where appropriate. Courteous interruptions when enough information has been obtained about a given point, followed by another question, will also keep the interview focused and make it possible to accomplish the interviewing task within a reasonable period of time.

There are patients, however, who will not be hurried. Their obsessive need to recall detail and to present all of it to the interviewer is so great that attempts to focus the interview fail to hasten the patient's account to any measurable degree. Impatience or anger on the part of the interviewer will only complicate the relationship and make matters worse. In such cases, it is best to relax, to accept the situation as gracefully as possible.

> The patient was a forty-year-old obsessive man who was describing the pressure of each job he had after leaving a somewhat subordinate position in a large industry for a series of executive positions with small, federally funded community projects. Midway through each such description it became apparent that the pressures were similar and the patient's symptoms were identical each time they recurred. In describing the third recurrence, the interviewer decided to interrupt.
>
> PATIENT: And then the stomach pains began again. First I began to notice that I'd get nauseated after breakfast—
> INTERVIEWER: (*Interrupting*) Were the symptoms the same as the first two times?
> PATIENT: Oh, yes. (*Goes on to recount them all, once again.*)
>
> The interviewer took a deep breath, settled back, and, glancing at his watch began to rearrange mentally the remainder of his day.

Another type of over-talkativeness is encountered in the patient who rambles. Often elderly, or simply garrulous, this patient does not behave as an obsessive patient does, but he seems to be poorly organized. With this type of patient, one should interrupt when the patient wanders away from the topic at hand unless the patient is in fact supplying information that appears indirectly relevant. Refocusing the patient's attention may be frequently necessary. There is still another type of very talkative patient whose chattering quality betrays his underlying anxiety. A friendly, reassuring, or supportive comment about the patient's evident anxiety is often sufficient to reduce it.

Since for many people verbal communication is a way of controlling and reducing the freedom of the other individual, there is a danger with some patients that the interview can become a battle of wills. To get the job done, and to reassure the patient that the interviewer is, in fact, capable of carrying out diagnosis and treatment, the interviewer should not allow control of the interview to slip into the patient's hands. On the other hand, an interview should be conducted sensitively enough that the patient does not feel dominated or over-controlled. Most patients respect a clinician whose manner suggests strength and self-assurance. But there are individuals who cannot stand the feeling of being subservient. This, in itself, need not pose a problem. But when such a patient cannot accept a relationship of mutual participation, the relationship can be a severe trial of patience for the clinician.

Not all over-talkativeness represents an attempt to dominate the other person. Some patients feel a kind of closeness when talking. They tend to be lonely individuals who cannot tolerate silence and feel that there is a bond between them and the other if someone is speaking. This is detectable by the interviewer, who will feel it as a "sticky," clinging kind of communication. Bed-ridden patients suffering from chronic disease will often make every effort to prolong interviews and keep on talking, fearing that the interviewer will go away.

The Seductive Patient

The patient has certain expectations of the clinician-patient relationship which play an important role in his interview behavior. He expects to have the source of his disorder found and corrected. He expects some degree of comforting or care, some reassurance, and a successful outcome. Sometimes the patient's expectations about the outcome are unrealistic, and no patient likes to hear that it may not be possible to help him.

Some patients may have unrealistic expectations of another variety. They may look for more than a professional relationship. Some may develop fantasies of an intimate personal relationship or even a love affair. And some may behave seductively with the clinician in an effort to make their fantasies come true. Usually such patients are hysterics, or they may be in a hypomanic or manic episode of an affective psychosis.

With the hysterical patient, or with the patient who has become attracted to the physician but who is not psychotic, such seductive behavior will rarely emerge in an open and undisguised way. But there are clinicians who, consciously or unconsciously, foster such unrealistic expectations about an intimate, non-professional relationship.

A special problem is posed for every clinician when he finds a patient of the opposite sex very attractive. Young physicians, in particular, may have to cope with their own feelings in response to such patients, though this problem is by no means confined to young people. Older clinicians whose personal or family lives are unsatisfying or in disarray may respond to an attractive young patient with sexual feelings and a desire to convert the professional relationship to a social one. It is important to recognize these feelings, to accept them as a natural response, and to keep clearly in mind that they cannot be acted upon.

In some instances physicians may be seductive by encouraging unrealistic expectations about prognosis. In a misguided attempt to create trust and confidence, one can become overly supportive or misleadingly reassuring. Overdone warmth can be seductive and stimulate fantasies of love or sexual relationships. The clinician should avoid such indirectly seductive behavior as telling his troubles to the patient and seeking emotional support from the patient. It is not wise to use pleasing the physician or nurse as a motivation for cooperating with treatment, as this may stimulate fantasies of personal reward for good behavior. Physical expressions of affection can be very seductive. And, of course, from time to time a clinician and patient do seduce each other, often with disastrous results for the personal lives and families of both.

When a patient is openly seductive or makes direct sexual advances the correct response is a firm, professional one. Without scolding or moralizing, the patient must be reminded of the limits of a professional relationship. If these steps are not taken, explosive complications may result.

The Angry Patient

Another trial of patience for the interviewer is posed by the angry patient. Anger can be a response to illness. There are people who ordinarily can tolerate delay in having their needs cared for but who become short-tempered and irritable when they are ill. They become angry, demanding, and highly critical of the physician or other health professional. One can read between the lines, in the patient's behavior, a communication of fear. The patient is saying, "I am afraid that there is something seriously wrong with me. Are you doing everything you can to help me?" When one feels unfairly attacked, it is a human response to react with anger. However, this will damage the relationship and greatly reduce the possibility of helping the patient. When the patient is angry, one should try to step back and examine what is happening. Warmth, appropriate reassurance, and an open recognition of the relationship of anger to fear is most likely to be helpful.

In other instances, the interviewer finds himself the target of an irrational angry outburst seemingly unconnected with him. Anger may be displaced from an unavailable target (spouse or employer for example) or from a situation which has just occurred in which the patient did not have the opportunity to express his angry response. For example, a receptionist may have handled the patient in a cold and abrupt manner and turned away without allowing him a chance to voice his anger. In the hospital, a patient may have been treated insensitively moments before by a technician, nurse, or orderly. A little time will permit the anger to subside. A comment like "I find it puzzling that you are angry with me" may uncover the true source of the anger.

Students sometimes become upset when they encounter an apparently irrational angry response from a patient they are about to interview. Sometimes the anger is ascribed by the patient to the fact that it is a student who is about to interview or examine him. This calls for an examination of the patient's anger with him. Here, a confrontation is the best way of proceeding. "You sound very angry" makes the patient's response the opening topic. Some patients, or their relatives, may insist that they are not willing to be interviewed by a student. At such a point, it is best to bow out gracefully and call for help from a staff member, supervisor, or resident physician.

Of course, there are also times when the clinician has provoked the anger himself. Brusqueness, sarcasm, moralistic comments, or attitudes of superiority easily provoke anger. This may be a matter of thoughtlessness or haste. Too often, doctors interview hurriedly because of time pressure. One should always examine one's own behavior before ascribing anger to some difficulty or personality trait of the patient.

Anger can be a defense against the threat of feeling closeness or warmth toward the interviewer. This response may be provoked by the interviewer's overly warm or seductive attitude, though it may be aroused in some patients by simple expressions of professional concern. If this is perceived as threatening by the patient, he may react with anger. The threat of feeling warmth or closeness provokes some people to anger in an effort to drive the other person away. Such patients can tolerate receiving help from relatively cool and reserved individuals.

There are individuals whose life style is characterized by anger. They are angry at everyone around them. Even in repose, their manner and facial expression communicate this. The chronically angry man or woman is always a difficult problem for the interviewer. Often his difficulties are related to his anger. The clinician must keep in mind that he is not the primary or sole target of this anger. Observation and the history of the patient should make clear that this is part of the patient's life style and that it is possibly related to the discomfort that brings the patient to seek help.

Aggressive behavior in general is often a means of dealing with a feeling of helplessness or a fear of surrendering to tendencies to be passive and dependent. Some people customarily handle their fear of becoming dependent by maintaining an aggressively independent stance and struggling to maintain control of every situation. For such patients, to become ill increases their fear of passivity and helplessness. They are likely to react with anger at being a patient. When a topic is introduced that touches on an area in which they feel inadequate or where they fear they have failed, they are likely to become angry and abruptly dismiss it. It is best not to push for information at this point. If the patient begins to feel that he can safely depend on the physician without completely surrendering his autonomy, he is likely to be willing to supply the information later.

The Paranoid Patient

Occasionally the clinician will encounter a patient who has a paranoid personality. Such individuals are chronically angry, suspicious, and distrustful, and they easily become convinced that some person or agency has a malign plan or design directed against them. They tend to brood, become depressed over real and fancied injustices, carry grudges, ruminate about wrongs which were experienced years before, and quickly assume that the clinician's intention cannot be trusted. Such patients may or may not be delusional, but in either case they are most difficult to interview. Any topic which arouses their suspicion, or provokes angry accusations, should not be pursued. Warm and reassuring behavior tends to be threatening to these patients and provokes more paranoia. It is best to maintain a friendly but cool and detached neutrality with paranoid patients. Tactful firmness, avoidance of angry responses to the patient, and consistency help to build whatever sense of trust the patient may be capable of feeling. Reassurance and support, on the other hand, which might be warmly received by most patients, is usually very upsetting to the paranoid patient.

A Note on Evasive, Indirect, and Embarrassed Patients

Sensitivity to the patient's experience in the interview dictates that one may not always proceed at once to the task of gathering data about the patient's present complaints and problems. When a patient shows evidence of evasiveness or indirectness, it is a natural tendency to push harder for information, to make one's questions more specific and more pointed, or to press for more precise and detailed descriptions. This is a mistake. There is usually some topic or concern that the patient must get out of the way first. Evasiveness or indirectness frequently means that the patient is ambivalent about talking about something, knowing that it would probably be helpful but fearing to speak openly. The patient may be embarrassed, feel guilty, or fear that something about to be revealed will not be kept in confidence. The skilled interviewer will, at this point, abandon the direct inquiry and shift to a discussion of the patient's behavior and apparent discomfort. A comment like "You seem to be having a great deal of difficulty talking about this" will often open a discussion of the source of the difficulty. After the discussion it should be possible to continue the inquiry with less reticence on the patient's part. Other patients have difficulty talking to anyone and will require somewhat more direct questioning and specific inquiries to elicit details than the usual patient.

The patient who states early in the interview that he'll be happy to answer the doctor's questions may appear to the inexperienced interviewer to be especially cooperative when actually he is frequently hoping to avoid certain areas of information. His is not a cooperative attitude. He is saying, in effect, "I won't volunteer a thing." Similarly, other patients, basically passive or dependent individuals, have great difficulty volunteering anything and prefer to be led, to be asked questions to which they will supply answers rather than to volunteer information. This is often experienced by the interviewer as demandingness, which is exactly what it is. If the clinical relationship continues, these patients are likely to become more and more openly demanding. It is important for the clinician to understand the reason for the demand and to maintain an appropriate distance. In this way he will be able to avoid becoming angry and possibly punitive.

Social Distance

The interviewing task is considerably more difficult when there is a great deal of social distance between clinician and patient. The problem lies on both sides. The patient's reservations, ability to trust, and ability to cooperate will be influenced by the attitudes he brings from his culture and his social class to the physician-patient relationship. The patient of low socio-economic status sees the upper-middle-class professional much as he sees all persons of a higher status rather than purely as a helping person. Similarly, the clinician, no matter how hard he may try to transcend this distance, will carry attitudes into the interview that reflect his feelings about the patient as a representative of his class or cultural reference group. The physician, nurse, social worker, or other health professional who interviews a patient must examine himself carefully for the ways in which his attitudes, prejudices, and values are preventing him from being, first and foremost, the patient's advocate and helper. He must also learn to correct for those attitudes, suspicions, and behavior that reflect the patient's social and cultural origins.

3   EMOTIONAL ASPECTS OF THE PHYSICAL EXAMINATION

If a well-conducted interview has preceded the physical examination, a relationship has been established. The physician is no longer a stranger but a concerned individual who is trying to be of help. The physical examination is one more step in the data collection process. Without such an interview, the physical examination is an invasion of the patient's privacy and may even be experienced as a humiliating assault.

Disrobing in front of someone else is usually done in intimate situations with a trusted person. "Naked" is almost a synonym for "defenseless." For this reason, the fully clothed physician must always be aware of the problem of shame, embarrassment, and feelings of inferiority that his unclothed patient may experience. He should permit the patient his dignity by seeing to it that he is properly draped. He should be polite, business-like, and not linger over especially emotion-laden areas like breasts, genitals, and rectum; but he should not be so swift as to suggest that *he* is embarrassed. Alertness to evidence of shame, embarrassment, and guilt feelings is most important. If such feelings appear to be upsetting the patient or interfere with the conduct of the physical examination, a discreet inquiry or confrontation can lead to a discussion of the patient's feelings and a reduction in their intensity.

For some patients, the physical examination provides an opportunity to be seductive. Appropriate professional reserve and the presence of a nurse or attendant usually suffice to forestall any overt attempts to make the doctor-patient relationship a sexual one, but the physician should be aware that his own behavior can stimulate erotic fantasies in certain patients.

The patient may also have anxieties about specific areas of the body. If these are not detected in the interview, they can easily be seen during the examination in the patient's remarks as a given area is approached. This gives the examiner the opportunity to gather more data and the patient a chance to bring his anxieties out into the open. A simple confrontation, such as "You sound like you're worried about your (heart, bowels, or other area approached)," will usually suffice to bring out the patient's concerns or fears. The principle is this: interview and examination are not clearly differentiated separate processes. The interview is still in process during the physical examination.

REFERENCES

1. Blum, R. H., *The Management of the Doctor-Patient Relationship.* New York: McGraw-Hill, 1960.
2. Lederer, H. D., "How the Sick View Their World," *Journal of Social Issues*, 8:4-15 (1952). Reprinted in E. G. Jaco, *Patients, Physicians and Illness.* Glencoe, Ill.: The Free Press, 1958, pp. 247-256.
3. Leigh, Hoyle, and Morton F. Reiser, *The Patient: Biological, Psychological, and Social Dimensions of Medical Practice.* New York: Plenum Medical Book Company, 1980.
4. Enelow, A. J., and M. Wexler, *Psychiatry in the Practice of Medicine.* New York: Oxford University Press, 1966, pp. 267-271.
5. Schwab, J. J., F. R. Freemon, R. S. Clemmons, and M. L. Scott, "Differential Characteristics of Medical Inpatients Referred for Psychiatric Consultation: A Controlled Study," *Psychosomatic Medicine*, 27:112-118, 1965.
6. Spitz, R., "Hospitalism: An Inquiry into the Genesis of Psychiatric Conditions in Early Childhood," *The Psychoanalytic Study of the Child*, 1:255-278, 1945.
7. Bowlby, J., "The Nature of the Child's Tie to the Mother," *International Journal of Psychoanalysis*, 39:1-23, 1958.
8. Engel, G. L., *Psychological Development in Health and Disease.* Philadelphia: W. B. Saunders, 1962.

9. Morgan, W. L., and G. L. Engel, *The Clinical Approach to the Patient*. Philadelphia: W. B. Saunders, 1969.
10. Ibid.
11. Ballis, G. V., L. Wormser, E. McDaniel, and R. G. Greneu, *The Behavioral and Social Sciences and the Practice of Medicine*. Boston: Butterworth Publishers, Inc., 1978.

5

EMOTIONAL AND BEHAVIORAL RESPONSES TO ILLNESS AND TO PATIENTS

1 THE SUBJECTIVE CLINICIAN

Just as patients react to clinicians and to illness with a variety of emotional and behavioral responses, clinicians respond to patients and to illness in a variety of ways. Yet the subjective clinician is often overlooked by those who train health care professionals. Part of being professional, after all, is moderating subjective responses to patients and to illness in the interests of patient care. Even so, subjective reactions do occur and they can be important. If they are not acknowledged and understood, they can interfere with patient care, as in the following example.

A thirty-five-year-old injured construction worker whose back pain had persisted longer than the expected length of time for a minor strain, was interviewed in the outpatient clinic of a teaching hospital. The clinician, a first-year resident, had just come from a meeting where his performance had been severely—and unjustly, he felt— criticized by a senior physician. The patient was also feeling resentful and complained bitterly about having to be examined one more time, and by a junior clinician at that. "What the hell can *you* add to my treatment?" the patient growled at the resident. "This is just another way of putting me off."

The clinician felt his gorge rising and impulsively said, "Look, you don't want to be here and neither do I." This so upset the patient that he got up and left. After that he refused to submit to any further examinations, saying that he didn't want to be scolded again.

It is obvious that if the clinician had been able to recognize and accept how angry he was before seeing the patient, the patient's remarks would not have sparked the clinician's outburst. As it was, the clinician perceived the patient's response as yet another personal criticism and immediately retaliated in a way that alienated the patient. Indeed, the clinician could have used his own resentment at being unjustly criticized to understand how the patient might be feeling about having to submit to an interview that he thought unnecessary. A clinician's subjective responses can also enhance his ability to understand and help patients.

2   THE CLINICIAN'S REACTIONS TO ILLNESS

Clinicians have an active role in responding to an illness, while patients often become passive and dependent. These differences nearly obscure the fact that illness, sooner or later, affects everyone.

Clinicians were far more aware of this truth in the past. Osmond[1] points out that the last forty years have seen a dramatic change in the pattern of illness in industrialized countries, with serious illness in the first thirty years of life becoming less and less frequent. Thus, medical students and young physicians today are much less likely to have experienced illness themselves in any significant way. Further, the fact that most ill people are now cared for within institutions rather than at home means that young clinicians are not as likely to know what it is like to be around people who are ill. In the past physicians tended to have a deeper appreciation of illness as a part of the life process.

Unfamiliarity with illness, added to the expectations of their role as healers, makes coping with illness potentially stressful for clinicians. The next sections will describe the most common reactions of clinicians to illness.

Anxiety

Illness can produce anxiety in the clinician as well as the patient. Sometimes this is realistic, such as the fear of contracting an infectious disease, making a mistaken diagnosis, or doing more harm than good when treating an illness. Today clinicians also have realistic fears about possible legal problems should the outcome be unfavorable.

Clinical practice is conducted in such a way as to diminish some of these fears. For example, it is standard practice to use certain precautions when treating patients with highly infectious diseases such as hepatitis. It is also common for clinicians to work together or to consult one another when the diagnosis is not obvious or the treatment carries significant risks. Sharing the burden of responsibility can go far toward keeping fear within reasonable limits.

Sometimes, though, these measures are not sufficient and an effort has to be made to identify the fear and bring it into the open. The problem is that many clinicians are embarrassed about their fears. This embarrassment can vary with the culture from which the clinician comes. As children, many were taught to "be a man" and "keep a stiff upper lip." All have been subjected to training that demands meticulous attention to detail and great control and, later, to role expectations of possessing such control. All of this mitigates against the clinician feeling comfortable admitting to his fears and anxieties, much less doing something about them. Sometimes, in an effort to avoid being overwhelmed by their own anxieties, clinicians may behave oddly or even insensitively toward their ill patients.

Helplessness. The paradigm for the anxiety experienced by the clinician because of feeling helpless is the situation of caring for a patient with a terminal disease, especially cancer. No other situation makes a clinician feel more helpless. The clinician knows that no matter what he does, the patient will not recover. The more committed the clinician is to curing patients, the more helpless he will feel when trying to treat the patient with an incurable illness. As with patients, this helplessness may be so intolerable that behavior designed to demonstrate the opposite is acted out.

A good example of this is the failure to provide adequate pain relief for a dying patient in an effort to avoid creating an addiction
to narcotics.

Clinicians must offer both compassion and expertise. The subjective feeling of helplessness and the anxiety it provokes are
sometimes the only means by which the clinician can identify with
the patient. To reject the lessons taught by such feelings is to
render oneself incapable of being genuinely compassionate.

Compassion may be a virtue that is expected of clinicians, but
very little time is spent helping them develop it. They are rarely
taught to identify and value those subjective responses that enable
them to exercise compassion, and they are almost never taught
how to use these responses on the patient's behalf.

A female medical student was assigned to obtain a history and perform a physical examination on a hospitalized patient. The patient
had consented to this and had been told not to divulge her diagnosis.
Upon meeting the medical student, the patient announced that she
had lymphoma. She then proceeded to frustrate the medical student
by avoiding the student's questions and refusing to have a physical
examination. Instead, the patient rambled on and on about the times
her children started school, went away to camp for the first time,
moved away from home, or got married. At the end of the allotted
time, the patient told the student, "Come by tomorrow and perhaps
I'll let you feel my spleen."

The student left feeling angry and a failure. The next day, when she
had to tell her supervisor about the patient, she was very embarrassed
to report that she had been unable to complete her assignment because the patient kept wanting to talk about her children going away,
so "finally I gave up and just listened."

The senior physician was silent for a moment, and the student prepared herself for the inevitable criticism. She was surprised, however,
when the clinician said, "It was good that you listened. Now, did you
hear what she was trying to tell you?" The student thought, and said,
"Well, she was talking about all the times she has said 'Good-bye.' "
"Exactly," her supervisor responded. "She is talking about the fact
that she is dying, and you may be the first person who has had the

time to listen. When you go back to feel her spleen, you might explore this further with her. If she is religious, you could ask her if she
would like the hospital chaplain to stop by. No one should be alone
at a time like this, and because you were able to 'just listen,' we now
know how we can help her."

When clinicians are not taught how to use their feelings on the
patients' behalf, they often believe that these feelings are dangerous and should be suppressed. The ways of escaping them are
avoiding the patient, overtreating the patient's medical problems,
acting with hostility, or rejecting the patient.

Avoiding the patient is probably the most common manifestation of anxiety about being helpless because it involves a simple
act of omission. The clinician who avoids his terminal patients is
often quite unaware of it. He just somehow never gets around to
spending much time with those particular patients, there being
so much else to do.

Overtreating the patient's medical problems is an act of commission, but it can be even more difficult to spot than avoidance.
This is because it is behavior that appears to be thorough and
dedicated. While the following example is not that of a dying patient, the heroic response to a medical problem as perceived by
the clinician had nothing whatever to do with the problem perceived by the patient.

A thirty-five-year-old man was observing the placing of a suture in a
small laceration that his four-year-old son had sustained. As the
needle entered the skin, the son cried out in pain and fear. The father
fainted. The family doctor hospitalized the father at once. No diagnostic interview was done, but a battery of laboratory investigations
was begun. All findings were negative. Though the patient protested
that his anxiety may have been the cause of the fainting spell, the investigation continued at the insistence of the family doctor. Finally,
a sternal puncture and bone-marrow smear was done. The smear
showed a few abnormal cells which might be considered indicative of
a very early leukemia. This accidental and somewhat equivocal finding was communicated to the patient, who then became markedly

anxious. The family doctor cited it, however, as a justification for thorough laboratory studies.[2]

Hostility toward and rejection of the patient can manifest themselves in many ways. A common example is by transferring the patient to someone else for care. When a terminally ill patient becomes depressed in the process of dying, for example, the primary physician may be tempted to transfer the patient to a psychiatrist for treatment of the depression. It would be more appropriate to view the depression as normal under the circumstances and to treat it as such.

Anothed kind of rejection is more subtle, as in the following case reported by Chessick:[3]

> I vividly remember a young man, dying of leukemia, who became acutely depressed after a visit from a team of physicians. This group of physicians consisted of the chairman of the hematology department, three residents, and half a dozen medical students who were making rounds on the hematology ward. After I sat with him for a while, the patient reported to me that the sum total of their discussion in his hospital room concerned the quality of the radio that he had brought to the hospital. The patient realized from this that they had given up hope on him . . .

Although all clinicians experience some sense of helplessness when caring for the terminally ill, there is actually a great deal they can do for patients. They can help them recognize and accept their own feelings. If a patient's depression and hopelessness are severe, psychiatric or pastoral consultation can be called for. These measures let patients know that the clinician is aware of the patient's feelings and is prepared to help him deal with them; that while there is nothing to be done about the illness, much remains to be done for the patient.

Depression

When a clinician's despair at the inexorability of illness and the limitations of medical care is turned inward, it is he who becomes depressed. This can lead to distortions in both perception and judgment. It is common to work longer hours and more diligently when one is trying to keep from being overwhelmed by depression. This makes a clinician feel more immune to criticism, whether external or internal, that might charge him with not trying hard enough. Unfortunately, it cuts off the clinician from sources of emotional support such as family, friends, and non-clinical interests. Thus, he may be psychologically isolated at the moment the depression breaks through his defenses.[4]

Like other depressed individuals, depressed clinicians often don't realize that they are depressed. The depression is usually first recognized by their colleagues. A sensitive peer can confront the clinician with a statement like "You've been looking kind of down lately," which gives him an opportunity to acknowledge and talk about his feelings.

When confronting depressed people, whether clinicians or patients, it is vital to remember not to accuse or blame them for feeling as they do. Even such apparently benign statements as "You shouldn't let it get you down" can be misperceived as criticism, as external confirmation of the worthlessness and inadequacy they already feel. The most supportive thing a colleague can do is to break through the depressed clinician's isolation and let him know that non-judgmental help is available.

Denial

There are some clinicians whose customary way to deal with frightening feelings or impulses is by never permitting them to enter their minds. The use of denial is reinforced by training that focuses exclusively on the patient's problems. This leaves the clinician with the implicit sense that his own feelings are unimportant, something to be ignored or repressed.[5]

The use of denial makes a certain amount of sense. No one likes to experience feelings such as impotence and despair. In addition, many consider these and other feelings to be unprofessional. Clinicians who use denial to cope with their feelings about illness and death are, by definition, completely unaware of doing so. Unlike depressed people, they don't appear to be sad or overwhelmed. Rather, they seem to be in complete control. But if one watches what they do, the opposite is often the case. These are the clinicians who are most likely to avoid patients whose illnesses cannot be cured, and who are most likely to over-treat medical problems.

For example, one of the most frustrating situations in clinical medicine is the patient whose illness eludes diagnosis. A clinician who cannot tolerate uncertainty tends to have very few patients with illnesses he cannot diagnose and treat.

A thirty-one-year-old woman began to experience spontaneous episodes of panic, rapid heart rate, chest pain, dizziness, and a fear of going crazy that would last ten minutes to an hour. Numerous visits to emergency rooms, family practitioners, internists, and allergists ensued; multiple laboratory and radiologic studies were done; but no serious medical problem was diagnosed. The patient then saw a neurologist, who heard her story, told her that she had multiple sclerosis, and needed to be hospitalized right away for further study. Alarmed, the patient said she wanted to think about it, went home, and called her family doctor. She asked him if he thought she had multiple sclerosis and, if so, why he had not told her this. The family doctor told her honestly that whenever a person has such serious and debilitating symptoms as she did, all sorts of diagnoses have to be considered. Tests are done to make sure the symptoms are not due to a common, life-threatening, or treatable illness. In her case, such causes had been ruled out. The next test was that of time, to see whether her symptoms would go away or evolve into a pattern characteristic of a fluctuating and chronic disease such as multiple sclerosis. "That's a relief," the patient said. "He sounded so certain, and no one else had even mentioned multiple sclerosis." The patient was later diagnosed as having Panic Disorder and was successfully treated with an anti-depressant medication.

Dealing with clinicians who use denial can be difficult. Feelings are very frightening to such individuals. The best way to help is through peer support and sharing. It can be helpful when a trusted colleague says something like "I don't know about you, but I really feel like a failure when I can't figure out what's wrong with my patient." Confronting a clinician's denial in a gentle, supportive way lets him know that others have these feelings, that they are to be expected under the circumstances, and that they need not be overwhelming.

Projection

As with some patients, there are those clinicians who deal with all perceived internal dangers through projection. They control fear by removing it from unknowable and potentially dangerous internal events to more controllable, more comprehensible external targets which they misperceive to be the source of the problem. In the extreme, the use of projection can result in frank paranoia, but this is uncommon among clinicians. Paranoid individuals usually do not elect to go into professions that involve a great deal of intimate contact with other people.

Even so, clinicians who are not adept at identifying their own problems may inadvertently project them onto patients, causing errors in both diagnosis and treatment.

A resident in obstetrics was married to a demanding woman who made him feel inadequate in many spheres, especially as a breadwinner and as a sexual partner. His work, however, was a consistent source of self-esteem, and rather than face the conflicts in his marriage, he dealt with them by taking on extra hours in an outpatient gynecology clinic. Here he found himself faced with a population of healthy young women whose main concerns centered on sexuality and contraception. He found their sexual concerns especially irritating. At times he dismissed their problems as trivial and would ignore their concerns. Other times he would attempt to counsel the women by forcing them to admit that they didn't really love their husbands or by persuading them that their expectations for sexual satisfaction were unreasonable. It was not until the head of the clinic had received a number of complaints from patients that the resident was confronted. After initially reacting by angrily saying things like "Well, you should hear the stupid things they want to waste my time with," the resident finally broke down and was able to see that the women he "counseled" were those who reminded him of his wife, and the problem he was attempting to solve was his own.

Earlier, the importance of compassion—the ability to feel as the patient feels—was discussed. This kind of identification provides information to the clinician that can be invaluable in caring for patients. There is, however, another kind of identification with patients that can distort information. In projective identification, the clinician's feelings are attributed to the patient. If the young resident in the above example had been treating young husbands with sexual concerns rather than young women, he might have assumed that his patients felt about their wives as he did about his. This assumption could well have resulted in the clinician being unable to hear what the patient was saying and treating the clinician's problem rather than the patient's.

3   THE CLINICIAN'S RESPONSES TO PATIENTS

Patients are more than containers for illnesses or bearers of interesting problems. Yet young clinicians often view patients in this way and may be dismayed when they realize just how complex patients can be. Some patients have disorders that are difficult to diagnose, don't respond to treatment, and are complicated by other disease processes as well as by social, financial, occupational, or emotional concerns. Patients also have personalities that must be considered if their problems are to be diagnosed and managed as effectively as possible.

When a patient and a clinician enter a room, two people also enter the room. The professional nature of their meeting, with its well-defined roles, may obscure this shared humanity but does not negate it. The people who are clinicians will have personal responses to the people who are their patients. Whether these responses are positive, negative, or indifferent, they are relevant information and need to be understood. There is nothing "wrong" with having feelings about patients, but it is possible to make mistakes when these feelings are acted upon impulsively or are not recognized.

A young psychiatrist had a psychotherapy patient who was a very attractive man a few years older than her. Without being aware of it, the psychiatrist began to change the style of clothes she was wearing to work, opting for clothes that were both more casual and more revealing than those she customarily wore. At the same time, she began to wear more makeup than she usually did. Her patient never commented on this, but he began to fail to come to appointments. One day a male colleague complimented her on her appearance and teasingly asked her who the new man in her life was. It was then that the psychiatrist realized that she was strongly attracted to her patient, that this was being manifested in her seductive appearance, and that the patient's discomfort with this might be why he had become so irregular about his appointments. When she returned to her usual, more formal mode of dressing, the patient began to be more regular about his appointments, although it took several months before he was comfortable enough to begin to speak openly with the psychiatrist about his problems with women.

Just as with patients, clinicians' attitudes toward certain patients can reflect previously learned attitudes. For example, many young clinicians feel awkward when interviewing patients who look like, act like, or are the same age as their own parents. Even though the clinician is the authority figure, in the interview situation he doesn't feel as though he is. He may even neglect to ask pertinent questions, such as those relating to the patient's sexual history, that seem too personal and somehow "wrong."

In other words, the interaction between clinician and patient often has emotional undercurrents and these can affect the clinician's interview behavior. Some of the more common responses that can pose problems are disrespect, arrogance, aloofness, fear, depression, anger, malice, prejudice, and seductiveness.

The Disrespectful Clinician

Disrespectful nicknames for patients are often used by young clinicians in an effort to come to terms with the hopelessness of some aspects of clinical work. "Alkies" (alcoholics), "whales" (obese people), and the acronym GOMER (Get Out of My Emergency Room) are examples of such terms. McCue[6] has observed that these phrases do not usually survive the training years, but the attitude can.

Disrespect can be shown by over-booking and keeping patients waiting, by not returning phone calls, or by having paraprofessionals do all the talking with patients in the cases of physicians and dentists. Many clinicians have the mistaken idea that the importance of their work entitles them to do things they would consider rude and thoughtless in others, as in the following example:

> A female physician was undergoing an amniocentesis in a large university medical center. She was apprehensive about the procedure itself, as well as about its results, as she was in a high-risk age group for chromosomal anomalies. After receiving genetic counseling from a nurse and an ultrasound examination from a technician, the obstetrician appeared. Without greeting either the patient or her husband (also a physician), the obstetrician grabbed the layer of fat on her exposed abdomen between his fingers and asked, "What's this, sweetie?"

The Arrogant Clinician

Physicians are the group of health professionals most likely to be labeled arrogant and to be resented for it. Inglefinger[7] maintained that a certain amount of authoritarianism, paternalism, and domination is essential for the effective practice of medicine, but he also pointed out that "the profession as a whole is affected by a brand of arrogance subsumed under lack of empathy."

The problem is often manifested by an inability to identify with the patient's needs and by cutting the patient off from genuine communication through the use of technical language and jargon. The patient's need to understand what is happening to him is a basic one. The use of jargon is out of place when talking with any but the most clinically sophisticated patients (e.g., other clinicians). Medical terminology they don't understand confuses patients and makes them feel stupid. They then have a difficult time asking relevant questions and following instructions.

If a patient genuinely wants to understand his condition but can't, the reason almost always is that the clinician is unable or unwilling to explain it. The difference between most patients and most clinicians, when it comes to understanding medicine and dentistry, is that clinicians have studied it and patients haven't. What clinicians know can be taught to patients if there is a willingness to use everyday language and to spend a little extra time.[8]

The Aloof Clinician

Many clinicians become aloof when they have to care for excessively dependent individuals. These are the patients whose demands for attention know no bounds and who are sure the clinician can fully meet their needs. At first these very dependent patients make the clinician feel special and powerful, but as time goes on these feelings often give way to exhaustion and exasperation. When the clinician fully comprehends the intensity of the patient's needs, he is likely to withdraw emotionally and become aloof.

Feeling a desire to distance oneself from a certain patient can represent useful information about that particular patient. The clinician who recognizes this feeling can then take measures to better meet the patient's needs while attending to his own. He can close interviews with words like "See you later" rather than "Good-bye" to let the patient know that the relationship will continue. In addition, it can help to minimize the patient's anxiety if the clinician lets the patient know exactly when the next visit will be, while discouraging unnecessary contact with the clinician in the meantime. This sort of interview behavior helps the patient learn that he is valued for his ability to cope, not for his propensity to cling.

The Fearful Clinician

Clinicians often have to deal with angry patients and angry families. Now and then there will be a patient whose anger is such that the clinician becomes afraid of him or her. The patient most likely to arouse fear in the clinician is the "entitled demander," described by Groves.[9] These patients are as needy as those dis-

cussed in the previous section, but they express their needs differently by becoming aggressive, obnoxious, and intimidating. They
frequently threaten litigation or withhold payment.

The clinician who encounters such a patient may feel bewildered by his hostility and demandingness, then angry and finally
afraid. These feelings can help the clinician understand the patient. Asking oneself "Why do I find *this* patient's anger so infuri-
ating? Why do I find *this* patient's threats and insults so frightening?" is the first step toward handling the situation constructively.
At bottom, the patient has legitimate needs and these can often be
met without compromising either the clinician or the patient.

It is best not to argue with these demanding patients but to
agree with them, to a tenable degree, by saying something that
will acknowledge their realistic needs and give some reassurance
that these will be met:

> I know you're mad about this and mad at the other doctors. You have
> reason to be mad. You have an illness that makes some people give
> up, and you're fighting it. But you're fighting your doctors, too. You
> say you're entitled to repeated tests, damages for suffering, and all
> that. And you are entitled—entitled to the very best medical care we
> can give you. But we can't give you the good treatment you deserve
> unless you help. You deserve a chance to control this disease; you
> deserve all the allies you can get. You'll get the help you deserve if
> you'll stop misdirecting your anger to the very people who are trying
> to help you get what you deserve—good medical care.[10]

Finally, it is important for clinicians to accept the fact that they
will not like every patient they meet. The guilt that can arise over
disliking the unlikable patient can fuel the anger and fear that
these patients produce. It is understanding and empathy, not affection, that clinicians need to give patients.

The Depressed Clinician

Certain kinds of patients can cause clinicians to become depressed,
just like certain kinds of illnesses. Generally these are not patients
who are seriously ill. Rather, they are patients who develop one
symptom after another and who never get better no matter what is

done for them. It is depressing to work with such patients, and the clinician's depression is a reflection of what the patient is feeling.

These patients are people whose emotional pains are experienced as physical symptoms and whose emotional needs are met by having someone treat the symptoms, and thus the patient, in a concerned and caring way. Such patients' needs are best met by an ongoing relationship with a clinician, and it is precisely this relationship that they are trying to achieve by their constant array of symptoms. Through this relationship they seek to develop a sense of completeness and self-worth.

What makes these patients so problematic for clinicians is that the clinician's goal is to cure the symptom. A cure is precisely what these patients do not want, for to them a cure means that the relationship will end. So long as a cure is the clinician's objective and continued illness is the patient's, their interaction will be frustrating and depressing to both. Often a patient's wish for a relationship is such that he goes from one physician to another, enduring multiple diagnostic and surgical procedures that have unsatisfactory results.

A patient whose symptom does not resolve itself with adequate treatment, one who develops a new symptom the moment an old one is relieved, or who presents a long history of unhappy relations with physicians needs to be regarded and treated differently from other patients. It is best for the clinician to proceed by sharing the patient's pessimism, agreeing with the patient that treatment might not be completely effective, and offering long-term relief of the symptoms rather than a short-term cure as the goal. This gives the patient a sense that his suffering is understood, that he may hold on to his symptoms as long as he needs them, and that the relationship will continue. This also establishes realistic goals for the clinician, who can then proceed to treat the patient's problems without having to be depressed about not achieving a cure.

The Punitive Clinician

There are some patients who want to die. They express this wish by relentlessly self-destructive behavior. These patients can cause their caretakers to vacillate between wanting to help them and wishing that they would just get it over with. When a clinician has such discordant feelings about a patient, he needs to proceed with caution. The wish to die is the patient's, not the clinician's. The clinician who fails to realize this, or even to acknowledge his own feelings, may behave in a punitive way toward the patient. While this may actually be what the patient wants, it is not good clinical care.

A fair percentage of these self-destructive patients are actually very depressed, and their depression may be treatable. But even if they are not depressed, or if they refuse to be evaluated for depression, they deserve the same empathic support due any patient whose illness is life-threatening.

Another kind of patient can arouse punitive urges in clinicians. Occasionally a patient turns up who reminds the clinician of someone who was harsh or cruel to him and against whom he could not retaliate. Now, in the form of this patient, the old enemy is at the clinician's mercy. If the clinician does not identify these vengeful feelings in himself, he may unwittingly cause the patient unnecessary discomfort or actually harm him.

The Prejudiced Clinician

Most people think of prejudice in terms of race, religion, and, more recently, sex and sexual preference. Actually, there can be many groups against which a clinician may be biased, some more subtle than others. All have to be elucidated if patients who fall into these groups are to receive the care they are entitled to. The more invisible a clinician's antipathy toward certain human groups, the more visible his failures will be at providing the best possible care.

For example, many clinicians are prejudiced against patients who have been identified as alcoholics or mentally ill and may go to great lengths to avoid them. As the following example shows, this avoidance can be dangerous for the patient.

A patient came into the emergency room of a county hospital stumbling clumsily and mumbling incoherently. He had a long history of alcoholism and chronic schizophrenia. The night before, he had wandered into the same emergency room while inebriated and the staff called the police to take him to the drunk tank. Upon seeing him again the next night, the medical staff sent him to the psychiatric emergency room (a separate facility) saying that he was drunk again and needed to be admitted for detoxification, even though they knew he had just been released from jail after being there over twelve hours and therefore could not possibly be acutely intoxicated. The psychiatrist found the patient to be somnolent and then stuporous and to have focal neurologic findings as well as evidence of recent, severe head trauma. It took the psychiatrist twelve hours, during which time the patient became comatose, to convince the medical staff of the need for immediate transfer to the main county hospital where there was a CT scanner to diagnose and neurosurgeons to treat what turned out to be an intra-cranial hemorrhage.

The Seductive Clinician

Almost all books on clinician-patient interractions include discussions of the seductive patient. This type of patient, as well as possible responses from the clinician, was discussed in Chapter 4. Conspicuously lacking in clinical textbooks, however, is any discussion of the seductive clinician—the clinician who does not keep in mind that sexual attraction to a patient must not be revealed or acted upon.

Perhaps it is easiest to understand this sort of behavior by considering two aspects inherent in the clinician-patient relationship. The first is that the clinician is in a position of power and authority relative to the patient. The patient depends on the clinician to look out for his welfare and therefore does not wish to alienate him. The second is the physical intimacy that is part of the relationship. The only other people who are permitted to touch the patient in such intimate ways are sexual partners. The only other people whom the clinician touches in such intimate ways are also sexual partners. The behavior of a clinician who does not distinguish clearly enough between a desire to please and sexual desire, or between physical contact and sexuality, can be understood—although hardly condoned.

Sexual contact with patients is always detrimental and never appropriate. It constitutes abuse of patients and is unethical. Sexual feelings toward patients that occasionally occur during the conduct of clinical work should be appreciated as normal. Almost all clinicians will eventually encounter a patient whom they find very attractive. However, if the clinician is concerned about these feelings or is afraid he might act on them, he would do well to discuss the matter with an appropriate person, such as a supervisor.

4   EMOTIONAL ASPECTS OF CLINICAL WORK

Clinical work is challenging but stressful. One major source of stress has been the expectation, on the part of both patients and clinicians, that health professionals will leave their human fallibility and frailty behind when they go into clinical work. No one can live up to this kind of expectation, but many clinicians regard their inability to do the impossible as failure. A feeling of failure can cause the clinician to behave in ways that can harm himself—such as taking drugs to control his anxieties—or his patients.

Clinicians are people. Each brings to his interractions with patients his own personality, talents, and susceptibilities. His subjective self will be as present in every interview as his professional and objective self whether or not he wants it to be or is even aware of it. Subjectivity can be an ally in clinical work when it is recognized, understood, developed and when necessary, compensated for. Subjectivity is the source of the clinician's compassion and empathy. It can be a liability if it is renounced.

Clinicians are not machines, and this is what makes them so valuable to their patients. While it is their capacity to be professionally objective that sets clinicians apart from the people they serve, it is their subjectivity that binds them to their fellow human beings.

REFERENCES

1. Osmond, H., "God and the Doctor," *The New England Journal of Medicine*, 302:555-558, 1980.

2. Chessick, R. D., "Biomedical Progress and the Physician's Approach to the Patient," *Psychosomatics*, 22:625-628, 1981.
3. Enelow, A. J., and M. Wexler, *Psychiatry in the Practice of Medicine*. New York: Oxford University Press, 1966.
4. Martin, M. J., "Psychiatric Problems of Physicians and Their Families," *Mayo Clinic Proceedings*, 56:35-44, 1981.
5. Gorlin, R., and H. D. Zucker, "Physicians Reactions To Patients," *The New England Journal of Medicine*, 308:1059-1063, 1983.
6. McCue, J. D., "The Effects of Stress on Physicians and Their Medical Practice," *The New England Journal of Medicine*, 306:458-463, 1982.
7. Inglefinger, R., "Arrogance," *The New England Journal of Medicine*, 303:1507-1511, 1980.
8. Baker, L., *You and Leukemia*. Philadelphia: W. B. Saunders Company, 1978.
9. Groves, J. E., "Taking Care of the Hateful Patient," *The New England Journal of Medicine*, 298:883-887, 1978.
10. Ibid.

6

INTERVIEWING CHILDREN AND PARENTS

1 INTRODUCTION

Effective communication in health care is based on accurately perceiving and transmitting verbal and non-verbal information, ideas, feelings, values, and concerns. In the care of children, such communication depends not only on the doctor's relationship with the child but also on his relationship with a variety of people who play a significant part in the child's life. Good care depends on the clinician's ability to develop personal relations of mutual trust with all concerned. The goal is a relationship that takes into consideration the best interests of the child while at the same time respecting the unique relationship between parent and child. Ideally, the relationship should be strong and should attend to psychological and social aspects of growth and development, as well as to physical health, and to the family as well as the child. It must provide the foundation other health care providers will depend on when the patient becomes an adult.

While the principles of interviewing children, their parents, and other informants are essentially those discussed elsewhere in this book, particularly in Chapters 2, 3, and 4 certain special considerations apply to the care of children. For one, there is the short attention span of children. Also, though an adult patient may be reluctant to seek help and is often apprehensive, the decision to seek medical help is virtually always made by the individual himself. A child, on the other hand, is usually brought to the physician by others. The child's level of understanding and emotional development will strongly influence his attitude toward the physician and his level of anxiety. Young children often react with more fear when "going to the doctor" than do adults, adolescents, or older children. If the parent is upset, worried, or anxious, the child will respond with anxiety. On the other hand, realistic, supportive parents can provide comfort and reassurance. The clinician-child interaction thus reflects important aspects of the parent-child relationship. The child's level of development as reflected in his communication affects the clinician's ability to deal with both the child and those responsible for his care, usually the parents. Verbal communication with the very young child can be difficult and is limited by the child's vocabulary and language, which may have a different meaning to him than it does to the clinician. Very young children use words in a concrete sense and do not understand symbols and abstractions, taking them literally. Adults must learn to understand the child's language and to express themselves in a way that the child will understand. Also, the capacity for auditory memory and the ability to process auditory information develop slowly during the pre-school years. When interviewing a young child, therefore, the physician should be brief and direct and use simple language.

The cognitive functioning underlying the verbal communications of a young child is worth considering. The two-year-old child views parents and, to a lesser extent, other adults as omnipotent. Fraiberg tells the story of a two-year-old girl who said to her father, "Do it again, Daddy," after watching the sun set.[1] The child's belief in the power of the parents must be viewed with respect, not with amusement. The child's physician, and other clinicians, share that power in the child's mind. The physician or nurse must recognize this and avoid stimulating potentially frightening fantasies. Two-year-old children feel that their own thoughts and wishes have the power of action. Furthermore, the very young child's difficulty in fully separating reality from fantasy makes it essential for the clinician to aid the child in distinguishing reality and recognizing the limits of thoughts and wishes. As the growing child's capacity to deal with reality and with the adult world increases, these considerations become less critical. Despite these limitations, one should communicate directly with the child, even the very young, and not restrict oneself to interviewing the parents.

> After listening briefly to the rather vague recounting of ill-defined but apparently acute concerns of a young mother who was not generally so unclear, the pediatrician turned to the three-and-a-half-year-old girl who was the subject of these complaints and said, "How do you feel today, Susie?" "Fine." "Your mother feels you're sick," the pediatrician declared. "What do you think?" "Daddy's away and Mommy's worried," Susie said without hesitation.

Words are not the only direct source of information. The child may communicate a great deal with facial expressions, movements, and other body language.

2   SOURCES OF INFORMATION

In caring for children, the physician may need several sources of information, depending on the age of the child and the nature of the problem. In virtually all instances, however, the child should be the primary focus of the physician's attention. Parents usually take part in the interview, although their importance as sources of information varies with the age of the child and the specific problem. In the very young, parents are the major source of information. With the older child and adolescent, however, it is best to obtain a larger proportion of information directly from the child himself.

Very often, the clinician needs informants other than the parents, particularly those from the child's school. The teacher and day-care worker occupy an important place in a child's life, playing roles that have no true adult counterpart. They may have almost as much contact with the child as do family members. They also have expectations in regard to the child's behavior, performance, and development. Children view them as powerful and, often, threatening. Though not always understanding, teachers often can provide skilled observations of the child's behavior and general functioning. However, the relationship between teacher and child can be so close that strong emotions, both positive and negative, experienced on each side may influence their judgments and their behavior.

3 SETTING OF THE INTERVIEW

Choosing an appropriate setting for the interview requires a developmental perspective. For example, the ideal setting for interacting with a two-and-a-half-year-old child is quite different from one appropriate for a sixteen-year-old. Adolescents may be uncomfortable in rooms designed for toddlers. They may avoid pediatric waiting rooms occupied by mothers and younger children. Physicians should interview adolescents in their private consulting rooms rather than in examining rooms. In the pediatric clinic or office, a small separate waiting area should be set aside for teenagers, or they should be scheduled separately.

Though the ideal setting is often not available, certain general characteristics can be sought. The room in which an interview takes place should help make the young patient feel comfortable. As with an interview room for adults, it should have privacy and be as quiet as possible. It should not appear fragile or formal. It should convey the message by its furnishings and the objects in it that the room is for children, not adults. It is useful to place certain fear-provoking instruments out of sight in cabinets or drawers. With the young child particularly, the clinician may well dispense with a white coat or uniform. Some very simple playthings are helpful, such as crayons, paper, a rag doll, picture books, or a toy truck. Other easily available items such as pipe cleaners and tongue depressors can also be used in play with the young child.

It is wise to spend some time alone with children, even young ones. Observations may then be made that would not be possible if the parents were present. However, one should not force a separation of child and parents. Parents should be advised that the child may react with apprehension if there is a possibility that he will be left alone with the doctor. They should be instructed to be supportive toward the child and not to leave the office or interview room until the child seems reasonably comfortable. If they are unable to leave, they should stay to the side, encourage the child to interact directly with the interviewer, and limit their communication with the child.

4   THE INTERVIEW PROCESS WITH CHILDREN

The Role of Observation

Since the communication of children, particularly the very young, is in large part non-verbal, much can be learned even if the child says nothing. One should begin by seeing the child in the waiting room, if possible. This is the least threatening and the most familiar-looking setting in the office or clinic for the child. Note the child's general appearance, dress, position in the room, and relationship to the parents. Is he close or at some distance from the mother, or is he with the father? Is he quiet or loud and disruptive? Is he clambering onto or clinging to the mother? If so, how does the mother respond to the child? Are the parents permissive, or do they display anxiety or strict control? How do the parents and the child communicate in the waiting room? These observations yield basic information about the child, the parents, and their relationship and provide important cues to be followed up in the more formal part of the interview. As is the case with all aspects of the assessment of a child, a knowledge of developmental norms and of the past developmental progress of the child is critical to the evaluation of the data obtained. Clearly, that which is appropriate at one level of development may be deviant at another.

When observing or listening to a child, one must be cautious in interpreting behavior or drawing inferences. It must be recognized that certain aspects of the child's behavior or speech may be quite specific to the immediate situation (i.e., the clinic or medical office), particular aspects of an acute illness, or the physician or other staff members.

Use of Toys in the Interview

One can obtain a wealth of information by watching a child play with toys. Look for the child's initial interests and then observe how these interests change; in other words, observe the play patterns. What types of toys interest the child—guns and tanks or dolls and baby bottles? These choices exemplify how toys provide a mode of expression for children. Lourie and Rieger[2] have listed several categories of behavior associated symbolically with different toys:

1. Relationship interests—dolls, puppets, play houses, animals
2. Motor control—cars and airplanes
3. Aggression—soldiers, guns, inflatable clowns, punching bags
4. Communication—toy phones and typewriters
5. Construction and destruction—blocks, puzzles, clay
6. Creativity—dolls, clay, painting and drawing
7. Constructive interests—clay and drawing
8. Hyperactivity—generally moving from toy to toy; playing with movement toys

Play with Other Children

It is always useful to observe how a child draws other children into his play. Does he play alone, oblivious of other children, or does he actively pursue the company of others? How does he react when other children barge into his play activities? Can the child share his toys and cooperate? What roles can the child take? Can he be a leader on one occasion and a follower the next? What is the level of sophistication of his play? Does he join in building complex models or does he enjoy more primitive activities, such as throwing sand and wrestling? These factors all reveal much about a child's social and emotional growth. Again, norms for the child's age are critical in assessing these data. Social relationships, choice of play material, and activities themselves change progressively as the child grows and develops.

Observations Regarding Growth and Development

A clinician can assess the physical aspects of growth and development at the same time that he makes the psycho-social observations just discussed. He can judge the degree of the child's neuromuscular maturation. Small and large muscle group functions, coordination, and range of abilities will be revealed in minor and major motor tasks. A formal examination may not even be needed. Also, the clinician can observe hand-eye coordination. Look for abnormal movements such as rocking, stereotypic motions, self-stimulation, and choreiform or athetoid movements. Note the development of the skeletal structure, looking in particular for spinal deformities or dysfunctions. Evaluate age-appropriateness of muscle strength and hand, eye, and foot dominance.

These observations are essential in planning health care for children. Students sometimes protest that they do not have time to spend watching children play. But if the examiner has time to learn to do a spinal tap for meningitis or to struggle with performing an adequate examination of a tympanic membrane, he should have time to observe a child at play. In most instances, the clinician's observations on the first or second visit can provide a starting point for a series of reassessments. Nurses and other health care workers can observe and record a child's behavior at play. School teachers and day-care workers can also easily observe the child's play and report their findings to the physician.

Observations of Older Children and Adolescents

So far, this chapter has dealt mainly with pre-school and school-age children. Non-verbal communication is equally important with older children and adolescents, although it may be less obvious to the observer. Body position, seating placement, and manner of dress are all modes of expression and avenues of communication, as they are with adults. In dealing with adolescents, a great deal can be learned by watching their interaction with parents. Indeed, the adolescent's description of these relationships is often misleading. Adolescents, who are usually struggling with conflicts relating to independence and self-definition, may verbally paint one picture while providing a very different one non-verbally. For example, a fifteen-year-old who verbally abuses his mother in a group situation may also sit very close to her, attend to her statements with a subtle eagerness, and maintain close eye contact with her. These observations would tend to suggest that the apparent hostility is superficial and the nature of the relationship far more complex.

Older children and adolescents may express their anxiety, their reluctance, or their hostility through silence, eye avoidance, slouching, and shrugging of the shoulders. Such resistance is particularly likely if the patients' problems center around behavior, school performance, or interpersonal relationships. Children with serious medical problems, acute or chronic, may appear tense and apprehensive, often with an anxious facial expression, clenched hands, and rigid posture.

Beginning the Interview

If the interviewer does not know a child and his parents, he should introduce himself fully, usually while observing the child and before proceeding to the examining room. It is better to defer discussing what you plan to do until privacy has been provided.

Initially, the child is likely to be apprehensive. A few friendly words or non-threatening questions such as "How old are you?" or "Do you have brothers or sisters?" may reassure the youngster. If the patient has been seen before, it is wise to acknowledge that you remember him with a reference to some prior interaction. Recognizing a recent or upcoming birthday is an excellent device when appropriate. In any case, a few moments of attention exclusively devoted to the child may help allay anxiety and minimize later communication difficulties.

Too often the interviewer talks only to the mother and does not bring the child into the conversation. This is a serious error. Early in the interview, the clinician should give the child an opportunity to talk about his complaints. The "menu" approach can help the child describe his problem. This approach originated in child psychiatry but is easily applied to other aspects of pediatric medicine. By providing a "menu" or a series of questions offering a number of possible responses in a creative and imaginative fashion, one allows a child to express his concerns and views about his illness. The "menu" concept does not imply a series of true or false or multiple choice questions. Rather, it is used to indicate a series of gently probing comments or inquiries into several aspects of the child's symptoms or life. The aim is to find topics for conversation or for other means of communication, such as play, which can be used to establish dialogue and eventual rapport.

These comments or questions may relate directly to the child's current symptoms, school or family life, play activities, friends, or perhaps to the child's appearance or a toy. With older children and adolescents, local social or athletic events or news items may be equally helpful. It is often useful to focus on certain pleasant aspects of the child's life in a friendly way.

An example of the "menu" approach follows.

DOCTOR: Let's see, Jimmy, haven't you had a birthday since the last time you were here?

JIMMY: Yes.

DOCTOR: Are you five years old now?

JIMMY: (*Nods*)

DOCTOR: How does it feel to be five? (*a very tough question for a young child*)

JIMMY: (*Shrugs and stares at doctor*)

DOCTOR: Do you like being five?

JIMMY: (*Nods*)

DOCTOR: Does that mean "yes"?

JIMMY: (*Nods again*)

DOCTOR: Does this mean "no?" (*shakes his head*)

JIMMY: (*Nods, smiling*)

DOCTOR: Oh, now we can talk. How do you feel today?

JIMMY: (*Shrugs and has puzzled expression*)

DOCTOR: Do you feel good?

JIMMY: (*Shakes head*)
DOCTOR: Do you feel sick?
JIMMY: (*Nods*)
DOCTOR: Do you feel real sick?
JIMMY: (*Shakes head*)
DOCTOR: Oh, I see, you feel a little sick. Is that right?
JIMMY: Yes (*very softly*)
DOCTOR: Do you hurt anywhere?
JIMMY: (*Nods*)
DOCTOR: Will you point to where it hurts?
JIMMY: (*Points to his ear*)

In this example, the doctor offers alternative answers as well as alternative modes of responding—that is, words, head movements, facial expressions, and hand gestures. He not only conveys an understanding of these modes of communication but also uses them to some extent himself. Thus, both in word and deed he gives the child permission to communicate.

The choice of words and their pronunciation, as well as complexity of sentence structure, are important in interviewing children. One must be understood but must not talk "down" to a child.

Children, of course, are supremely self-centered and often inhabit their own fantasy world. Only gradually do they become aware of the complexities of life and the realities of daily living.

It is important, particularly in difficult situations, to determine which world the child is in and how one may approach it to give the child the care he needs. This point is demonstrated by the following experience:

The patient was a small boy from whom neither the physician nor the nurses and house staff could get a blood sample. The child would fight, scream, and carry on hysterically. After fighting wildly with the boy, they gave up their valiant but unsuccessful effort and let him rest. Later, the physician returned and asked the boy why he made such a fuss. This little boy responded by saying he thought they might cut off his penis! With this revelation, the physician had the solution to the problem. The boy was encouraged to hold his penis with one hand while blood was taken from the other free arm. The sample was obtained with little trouble.

Recognition of the child's position on the spectrum from reality to fantasy resolved a difficult problem.

Most experienced clinicians can give similar examples of imaginative approaches used to solve problems. Such approaches to the interview can allay the anxiety of potentially uncooperative children and can also enhance the communication and understanding of cooperative children.

A three-and-three-quarter-year-old girl was brought to the clinic by her foster mother because of the child's bizarre behavior. Five months earlier the child had been hospitalized as a result of child abuse in which her right buttock had sustained second- and third-degree burns, together with other injuries. She was offered a selection of toys. She was able to express her anger, resentment, and other feelings during play with a "play house" in the clinic. One example of this was when she taped up the stove in the kitchen of the playhouse. This was a daily ritual. She also began to verbalize her feelings by talking into a toy telephone. Up to the time of the telephone play, this child had not been able to talk about the events associated with the burning incident.[3]

The Family History

The history of the immediate family should begin with data about the parents' health. A general inquiry should be made first, using an open-ended question referring to family health first. The current health status and major health history of the grandparents and all siblings should be obtained in all instances. Any unusual health history in other members of the family should also be noted and may indicate the need for establishing a detailed family pedigree.

If the family is new to the interviewer or clinic, the mother's history should be obtained in considerable detail, beginning with her own growth and development, the onset of her menarche, her first marriage, her first pregnancy, and each pregnancy thereafter. The information on pregnancies will vary somewhat with the specific problem at hand, but in general it should include a brief chronological statement about the mother's health during the pregnancy, its duration, the date of delivery or other termination, the birth weight of the infant, immediate postpartum problems, and information about the postnatal course of the baby. Inquiry into contraceptive practices is useful, as this will often provide information as to the planned or accidental nature of the pregnancies. An appropriate medical history of household contacts should also be obtained.

Family Histories in Genetic and Growth Disorders

In collecting diagnostic information about a child, the family history is often of special significance because of the frequency with which genetic disorders are first encountered in children. Also, the early determinants, or precursors, of many adult diseases can be ascertained during childhood. If there is any reason to suspect a significant familial or genetic disease pattern, it is helpful to develop a full family pedigree. This should include, as a minimum, the ages, present health status, and causes of significant morbidity or mortality for the siblings, parents, parental brothers and sisters and their offspring, grandparents, and great grandparents. If any significant pattern of illness or of a genetic trait is noted in developing the pedigree to this extent, one should then explore the same information for the siblings of the grandparents, their offspring, as well as siblings of the great grandparents and their offspring. It is often not only time-saving but also valuable for clear recording and analysis to make a diagram of the pedigree with the informants at the time the history is taken. In this way, one can attach correct names to each individual in the pedigree and be sure of the exact relationships of the people involved. This is of great assistance when additional family history is obtained as subsequent interviews.

Additional history should be obtained in the case of patients with growth disorders or nutritional disturbances. The stature and body habitus, as well as socio-economic class and ethnic origin, should be determined for as many family members as can be identified. A history in comparable detail is useful in many other disorders, such as diabetes mellitus, malignancy, and allergy, in which there may be genetic factors.

Past Medical History

The pregnancy from which the child patient was born is of great significance. One should inquire about the mother's prenatal care, its source, frequency, and the stage of pregnancy when it was begun, as well as the character of the labor and delivery. Not only will significant medical information be obtained, but this line of inquiry can be fruitful in eliciting parental attitudes toward sexuality, health care–seeking behavior, and family life in general. Frequently parental attitudes toward individual children have their origin in the circumstances surrounding the pregnancy from which a particular child was born. Such information is often useful in understanding complex behavioral patterns later in life.

The newborn and infancy period of the patient should then be evaluated in chronological order. It is helpful to obtain information on the birth weight and neonatal course of the patient. The specific details of this are frequently not available for children in large families or for older patients. The duration of hospitalization at the time of birth, both for the infant and for the mother, may be an indicator of the presence of neonatal problems and may prompt an examination of the hospital records.

At this point, the history can be further developed chronologically from the neonatal period up to the patient's present age, or a series of specific inquiries can be made about nutrition, illnesses, accidents, hospitalizations, immunizations, personal habits, and general development. The choice of one of these two approaches, or of a combination of the two, is usually made at the time of the interview and is based on the interviewer's sense of what problems seem most pressing. In either case, information should be obtained in each of the above-noted areas in most situations. In infancy, it is important to know if breast feeding was attempted, for how long, and with what success. The types of feeding formulas that were used, how frequently they were changed, and for what reason also should be determined. The immunization history is most easily obtained while discussing infancy. Information about later booster immunizations should not be forgotten.

Illnesses, poisoning, accidents, and injuries are subjects of importance in the pre-school child. Since this is the period when weaning, toilet training, mealtime behavior, and bedtime behavior are established, information on each of these experiences should be sought. These areas may prove to be highly sensitive. Tact and sensitivity are called for in obtaining this history. The facts about these behaviors are important, but even more important are the parental concerns and attitudes toward their establishment.

Entering school begins another period of transition for the child. His age and the circumstances under which he began school should be determined. The school child's learning experience, school progress, and the changing character of his relationships with siblings, parents, peers, and adults may be points of significance. The problems presented by adolescent patients are discussed later in this chapter.

Mental Status Examination of the Child

It is usually neither necessary nor appropriate to conduct a formal mental status examination with a child. If the clinician carefully observes the child's behavior, paying attention to both verbal and non-verbal communication, he will gain a great deal of information. Does the child display a preoccupation with his own thoughts? Is the content of his thought and fantasy out of keeping with his developmental level? Does he have obsessive thoughts or display compulsive or repeated stereotypic behaviors? Is his emotional tone appropriate? Does he have the capacity to experience a range of emotions? Does he have particular fears? How does he deal with stressful situations?

The clinician can assess cognitive functioning by attending to the child's awareness of the current situation and his understanding of it. Can he concentrate and attend to questions? Is he aware of time, place, and person? Is his memory active and accurate? The child's use of words, his capacity to conceptualize, and abstract knowledge he has gained at home and at school serve as guides to his intellectual functioning. The clinician can assess the child's judgment through play, stories, or hypothetical play situations. The child's ability to relate to the examiner, other staff, and parents provides useful information regarding the interpersonal aspects of his life.

Interviewing the Adolescent

The adolescent patient requests help directly from a physician at times, and at other times help is requested indirectly through the parents. Sometimes, however, the contact is made against the wishes of the adolescent. In each of these situations, one would expect the interview to proceed differently, but this is not always the case. Whether or not an adolescent wishes to have help, he may be reluctant to reveal embarrassment and apprehension to adults. For some teenagers, the idea of continuing to see the same physician they saw as "mere children" is distasteful. They may associate that person too closely with the past and with their parents. On the other hand, some adolescents would rather settle for the familiar, with all its disadvantages, than risk the unfamiliar.

At times, the most useful interaction with a teenager can be an open discussion of the possibility of his seeing someone else. Even in a family practice, recognition that the adolescent may want his own doctor is appropriate and reassuring. "I wonder if you have thought that maybe you're outgrowing me," opens up the subject in a non-threatening way. The physician and adolescent patient can discuss this matter on subsequent visits and may reach a decision only after some time.

Adolescents do pose problems for parents, school personnel, and health care professionals. They are often mindless of health risks or, conversely, may be almost hypochondriacal in their concerns. Their fluctuations in mood, values, and directions are frequent, and though superficially this may appear to be of little concern to the teenager, these mercurial changes are perplexing, frustrating, and worrisome to parents. One must remember that part of adolescence is uncertainty about oneself, one's relationship to others, one's goals, and one's place in society. The physician, as well as parents, can provide some external sense of consistency and predictability. It is best to maintain an adult stance in speaking and interacting with an adolescent. "Playing" a peer role and adopting the child's language usually is not convincing.

5 INTERVIEWING PARENTS

Interviewing the Child's Mother

The mother plays the major role in meeting her child's health care needs. She can provide a wealth of information.

The clinician must recognize and appreciate the parents' ability to make numerous decisions every day about their children's health problems with no help at all. He should also give the parents due credit for recognizing a problem that exceeds their ability to solve and acting accordingly to seek advice about the child for a variety of problems, some of which are not "medical." Korsch[4] suggests that many physicians refuse to deal with any but medical problems because they feel they have no expertise in solving problems in other areas. In her view, "If an interview is conducted skillfully, empathetically [sic] and non-judgementally, it is not rare to discover that no decisions are required of us after all. If we find how the mother feels about a problem, what she's done about it and how it has worked, in most cases she will lead herself and us to the solution." If the interviewer is not open to the variety of questions and concerns that parents have, they may not mention them at all.

Ideally, the doctor's contact with the mother should begin before the birth of the child. Clinical interviews will indicate which patients are at risk for medical and psychological complications. A teenage girl forced to marry because of pregnancy will certainly have to cope with significant stress. The patient who cannot afford another child faces a situation frought with worry. A woman pregnant for the first time, who has never cared for a child, will fear the prospect. A woman with a past history of serious medical or mental illness always fears a recurrence of problems during pregnancy. The list could go on, but the goal remains the same: to maximize the chances for good prenatal care, a normal delivery, and successful postnatal adjustment. Thus, it is important to explore the mother's feelings about the pregnancy. One should encourage her to talk about how she feels pregnancy will affect her life and what she expects of motherhood. Whom can she depend on for support? How does she view her husband and her family's role, and how will these relationships change? The clinician and patient should explore issues concerning sexuality, body image, and marital relationships. What are her hopes and dreams, and what are those of her husband for the child? How do she and her husband feel about discipline? How will they make decisions? These are all questions that a physician should encourage a pregnant woman to ponder and discuss. If possible, the physician should become acquainted with the father-to-be and discuss all these issues.

Two areas in the parents' histories are of particular importance. The first is the family health history and genetic history of both parents. The second is the experiences of both parents with their own parents. What were their childhoods like? Were their parents warm and giving or distant and rigid? Was either parent exposed to abuse? By addressing these questions the physician and parents take the first step in preventive medicine and open the door to a more firm, effective parent-child relationship.

Parents who seek child care often do so after utilizing all other possible modes of intervention. They often bring the sick child to a clinic with apprehension and anxiety about the child and themselves. A woman may feel inadequate as a mother because she feels her child might have become sick as a result of her negligence. She may also feel inadequate because her attempts to deal with the problem have failed. The following case illustrates this point:

A young mother gave birth to a child with congenital heart disease. The baby died after a year of life that required the mother's most vigilant care. Subsequently, the mother was seen at a family practice clinic with her other children. She was found to have symptoms of gastrointestinal dysfunction, the "irritable bowel syndrome." Endoscopy and barium studies were performed but were not diagnostic. She had a great deal of guilt about the death of her child, and was filled with despair and a sense of helplessness. She blamed herself for what she believed was poor care of the child. She felt that she had a serious, undefined defect within her or that she had done something disastrously wrong during the pregnancy which had a lethal effect on her child.

A child needs love and support from his mother. The mother, too, has needs that are fulfilled by the child. For these to be met, the child must respond to the mother. The mother must be able to feed the baby and see him respond appropriately with sounds, smiles, and speech. If these responses are not forthcoming, she may feel frustrated, disappointed, resentful, or even angry. Lack of response from the child poses a threat to the woman's confidence in her ability to mother and may inhibit her further maternal development. Autistic or emotionally impaired children, children with congenital anomalies, and children with serious chronic illness can be stressful to their mothers in this way. These are considerations for the clinician in working with the mother. What methods has she used to take care of her child? What things worked? What things did not get a response from the child?

In discussing these issues, the clinician should tell the mother about various ways of caring for her child and the reason for each. Mothering does not come naturally to every woman. It is important to learn the strengths that each mother has, reinforce them, and help her utilize them fully.

Mothers' attitudes toward their children have many determinants. The mother's own childhood experiences with parents and family obviously have a great impact on her attiudes and behavior toward her children. The small child who wants to run around freely or the teenager who argues about frequency of dating and questions limitations on staying out late rekindles memories of past experiences and conflicts. These, in turn, color the parent's present attitudes and decisions. As consultants for the family, health care workers should recognize their own biases and be able to help family members see and interpret theirs. It is essential to approach the mother and father in a non-judgmental fashion. Instead of asking "Do you spank your children?" it is more effective and less threatening to phrase the question as "Do you sometimes find it necessary to spank the children?" The question "Do you ever get angry at him?" implies that some parents do not get annoyed with their children. It may heighten a parent's apprehension, provoke guilt, and create suspicion of you. "What does he do that makes you angry?" conveys a non-judgmental attitude about anger, although it carries the message that the child has done something wrong, which is, perhaps, a premature judgment. "When do you feel angry with him?" is even less threatening and can be a useful inquiry in that it neither condemns nor approves of this natural response. Remember that parents and children do not have full control over their emotional responses. They often need support, approval, encouragement, and guidance about their responses. Physcians and health care workers, since they are generally regarded as knowledgeable about parental behavior, are in a good position to provide this.

Interviewing the Child's Father

Changes in women's place in society have had an impact on health care, particularly on the father's role in child care. Fathers are now taking a larger part in child care and should be encouraged to participate in prenatal planning. In many hospitals, they are encouraged to be present at the delivery. This participation should continue into the postnatal care of the child, including the interviews of routine well-baby visits. The father should be encouraged to actively participate in the care of the newborn. Clinicians should elicit his observations and concerns during times of illness. In this way, the father grows closer to the child. A closer alliance between parents is also promoted, which will assist them to be more mutually supportive in times of stress. Mutual support and participation of both parents is required for the success of any treatment plan.

Special problems in interviewing parents arise when a child has a serious or chronic illness or disability. This always causes disappointment and preoccupation with the child and his problem. These unpleasant and troublesome emotions may be reinforced by frustration, misunderstanding, and shattered hopes in the process of seeking help. Such feelings may interfere with the effort to obtain a medical history. The physician must deal with them by encouraging their discussion before proceeding with the history. A cautionary statement is in order here. Recognition that parents may feel angry about the quality of care provided in the past should not include agreement that the care was inadequate.

Conflicts within the family, particularly between parents, pose special problems. The child's physician may be subtly and perhaps unwillingly drawn into taking sides with one or another parent in a situation where the child is simply the battlefield for other marital conflicts.

> A young mother proclaimed to the doctor that she was "sure" that he, too, felt her three-year-old son was too young for nursery school. The doctor asked if there was some concern on her part. The mother immediately denied it. A moment later she asked, "How do you feel about it?" The doctor did not answer but suggested she describe her feelings. He then learned that she was very anxious about the boy's going to nursery school, but her husband was exerting great pressure on her to send him because "the boy needed to get away from her." A family conference was arranged.

6 SPECIAL PROBLEMS OF INTERVIEWING CHILDREN

The Care of the Seriously Chronically Ill Child

Interviewing the chronically ill child should go beyond the illness itself to the patient's ability to cope with it. Like other children, children with leukemia, diabetes, or heart or kidney disease need to be loved, to be wanted, and to have friends. They want to go to school like well children. The physical and social limitations imposed by illness and its treatment may seem catastrophic to the child. In addition to the medical needs created by illness, such as dietary restriction and daily injections, the clinician must also consider the psychological and social needs of the chronically ill child. The young child whose identity is uncertain or the teenager who is constantly in turmoil may need support to buttress his self-confidence. Thus, the interview may be not only diagnostic but also therapuetic. The emotional and interpersonal life of the child may be difficult to address, but it must be explored. In particular, one must be alert not to create a dependency that may undermine medical management.

Health care workers who care for children with acute, life-threatening illness must maintain a measure of professional reserve, for clinicians can have strong emotional responses to sick children that may hamper their effectiveness. But when the distance between the physician or nurse and the patient becomes too great, the child's emotional needs will not be recognized. This can create problems in caring for the child later.

The risk of developing such a close relationship with a chronically ill child during the protracted course of treatment that it becomes difficult to maintain appropriate objectivity is greatest in such illnesses as leukemia, diabetes, hemophilia, and renal failure with dialysis. Treatment may last many months or years, and the development of feelings of closeness with the patient is almost inevitable. The health care worker comes to feel like a member of the child's family. This may lead him to project onto the patient or his family feelings that are inappropriate, arising from the clinician's own childhood or present family. One must be alert to the danger of such tendencies toward over-identification with the child. Introspection and self-awareness are important aspects of professional growth and result in better medical care. The clinician must take time to evaluate his own personal needs. An appropriate question is: Whose needs are being satisfied in caring for the patient?

Child Abuse

Child abuse and neglect is an increasingly common problem. Few situations are as likely to arouse feelings of anger, hostility, and frustration among health care professionals, and yet yielding to such emotions will reduce one's effectiveness in this delicate, difficult matter. Because of the serious and possibly life-threatening danger for the abused child, the clinician must employ great sensitivity in dealing with both the child and his parents. The ultimate objective must be protection of the child.

In interviews where child abuse is an issue, the interviewer must present most questions thoughtfully and carefully. Open-ended questions allow the child or parent the opportunity to present his version of the facts. A picture of the pattern of family relationships will emerge. The interviewer should seek to identify the forces that bind the child and adults toegther, as well as the forces that make life together difficult for them. A non-threatening, non-judgmental attitude is essential in obtaining the trust of the child and the parents. Parents who abuse their children commonly have low self-esteem. They often have unmet childhood dependency needs of their own. They may themselves have been abused as children. In general, they are likely to have experienced an unsatisfying relationship with their own parents. They strongly resist child-rearing advice, guidance, or counseling, for they usually expect criticism of their shortcomings.

One must take care not to act on the basis of superficial information or premature conclusions. From a psychological point of view, the origins of child abuse may not reside exclusively in the parents. Children can provoke abuse by vulnerable adults. Children may also be quite attached to abusing parents. It is important not to identify yourself primarily with the child. Parents might construe this as competition and consequently feel threatened. The clinician should give the parents an opportunity to vent their anger and frustrations. If a therapeutic alliance can be formed and strengthened during the first diagnostic interview, follow-up interview and intervention by agencies, as well as other treatment approaches, are more likely to be successful.

Behavioral and Learning Problems in School

School problems of children are frequently the reason parents bring children to the physician. Aggressive or otherwise disruptive be-

havior, withdrawal, and learning difficulties are among the most
common of these problems. In such cases, the child often feels that
he has been "caught" and will be punished. Consequently, the
child approaches the interview with a great deal of hostility. The
child with learning problems often feels that he has failed. He may
have little self-esteem. Some children may try to cover a sense of
inadequacy with defensive bravado, trying to blame the school or
other outside forces for their failures.

In any case, one must bear in mind that school is a large part of
a child's life. Much of a child's sense of self-worth and most of his
social relationships revolve around school. Children with school
problems also have problems with other children, who will often
have teased or shunned them. Peers may also reinforce inappropriate behavior, which in turn may intensify a child's conflicts with
school authorities and parents. Very often such children see adults
as punitive rather than helpful. These feelings will interfere with
the establishment of rapport with the interviewer.

Children with school problems usually see themselves as inadequate, friendless, and different. Interviews that focus solely on their
problems and failures may be very demoralizing to them. A search
for an area in which a child feels good about his performance or
behavior can be very helpful in establishing rapport. If school work
itself is largely a problem, can the child run fast or sing well? Has
he trained his pet dog, or can he successfully repair his bike? As is
so often the case, support and inquiry must go hand in hand. The
physician must avoid behavior that the child considers stereotypic
for all adults. He must not judge, criticize, or present platitudinous
"pep talks."

7 CONFIDENTIALITY

Almost inevitably, children and adolescents have certain "secrets"
that they withhold from their parents and often from other adults
as well. These secrets may be of considerable importance when
they reflect emotional, interpersonal, or social problems. The content may vary to some extent, depending on the child's age and

the nature of his problems. A young child may keep a frightening fantasy to himself, while an older child or adolescent may wish to hide some proscribed behavior. The child with an obsession may not divulge his thoughts to avoid being viewed as "crazy," while the anxious child may try to hide his fears.

Similarly, parents may have secrets that influence their behavior and emotional responses. A recognition of these secrets is valuable in understanding a clinical situation and may provide the essential key.

An eight-year-old girl had been referred to a child psychiatrist by her pediatrician because her school work was declining. She seemed unhappy and apathetic. Her brother, three years younger, was very aggressive, and this also concerned her parents.

The parents described bland family interactions. They both seemed to have difficulty remembering details. They admitted trying to placate their children with empty promises, fantasies, and "white fibs."

The child appeared depressed. Both directly and in her play she expressed a sense of loss and apprehension about future loss. She also felt her parents could not be believed.

The consultant discussed his findings with the parents and indicated that the symptoms seemed clear, but the factors underlying them were less so. Hesitantly, the parents admitted that they had been considering divorce for some time and had not been "living as man and wife" for almost two years.

When this was later discussed with all family members present, the girl said she had been suspicious of this but was afraid to mention it because "no one would talk about it."

This case example illustrates two important points: first, that "secrets" may be critical to understanding a family problem and, second, that people often know and respond to "secrets" although they do not talk about them.

The child's confidence in the clinician, allowing him to reveal these secrets, is a responsibility that must not be taken lightly. The physician may tell his young patient that the parents must be informed of his opinion and recommendations but that it is not necessary for all the details to be divulged. One can say, "Unless it would be harmful to you, I will keep the secrets you tell me. If I feel I must tell your parents, I will tell you so."

Although the importance of confidentiality is recognized for the adolescent patient and is likely to be handled as with adults, one must not forget the importance of privacy for the school-age and pre-school child. Even the very young deserve that degree of respect for their integrity. It is often no less important for them than for older persons. This holds true even though children seem to expect that the doctor will report to the parents much as a teacher or baby sitter would.

Although it is important to provide an opportunity for the young patient to talk privately with the doctor for part of the interview, it is equally important to have joint meetings with the child and parents. This is particularly so when findings, opinions, and recommendations are discussed. The physician should not be a "pipeline" between child and parents.

8 SUMMARY

In this chapter we have tried to provide an understanding of the skills and attitudes needed for interviewing young patients and their families, the most appropriate settings for the interview, and some of the common problems. Health care of children is associated with problems not encountered in the care of adults. Among these are a lesser capacity to communicate, the dependent status of children, the effect of your care on their ultimate emergence as adults, the constant developmental changes, and the role of children in our society. Much time and effort may be required in interviews with children and their parents, but they can be among the most rewarding in all of health care. Professionals who work with children have the unique opportunity to see their young patients gradually become adult members of the community. During this time, they can play a significant role in the child's growth and development. If their task is done well, they will have helped the young adult acquire a sound foundation for a life that will be healthy, both physically and mentally.

REFERENCES

1. Fraiberg, S., *The Magic Years*. New York: Charles Scribner's Sons, 1959.
2. Lourie, R. S., and R. E. Rieger, "Psychiatric and Psychological Examination of Children," in S. Arieti (ed.), *American Handbook of Psychiatry*, second edition. New York: Basic Books, 1974-1975, vol. 2, p. 1.
3. P. A., and J. F. McDermott, Jr., "The Treatment of Child Abuse. Play Therapy with a 4-Year-Old Child," *Journal of Child Psychiatry*, 15(3):430-440, 1976.
4. Korsch, B., and E. F. Aley, "Pediatric Interviewing Techniques," *Current Problems in Pediatrics*, 3:1-42, May 1973.

7

INTERVIEWING THE OLDER ADULT

1 INTRODUCTION

Currently 11 percent of the population of the United States is over the age of sixty-five. It is predicted that by the year 2020 that percentage will rise to almost 20 per cent. People are not living longer; rather, more people are reaching old age, and the complexion of our society is changing as a result. Health professionals of all types will be spending more time caring for older persons.

Illness is much more common in the elderly, though it should not be accepted as "normal." In fact, most older people live healthy lives and many rarely see a physician. Nonetheless, the elderly consume more health care dollars than any other segment of the U.S. population, accounting for 33 per cent of all health care expenditures.[1] The elderly often have multiple chronic medical problems. When acute illness occurs, it is almost always superimposed on an underlying disorder. Although 80 per cent of the older population have at least one chronic condition,[2] from vision impairment to heart disease, when asked to rate their personal health 85 per cent reported being in good or excellent health.[3] This figure probably reflects some denial as well as some capacity to adapt to age-related conditions. Because of the prevalance of multiple problems and frequent denial of these problems, effective interviewing and an accurate history play a crucial role in the care of the elderly.

A point to be remembered is that the elderly grew up in a very different age. They have experienced world wars, depressions, the emergence of rapid communication and transportation systems, and the death of many of their close friends and family members. Many of them see hospitals as way stations on the path to institutionalization or even death. They are survivors and may be fiercely independent. This attitude sometimes makes their care difficult.

But the elderly are also products of the here-and-now. They watch television, read advertisements, and talk to friends about "miracle cures." They, too, are subject to the myths of our society: young is beautiful, old is unattractive; once old, one must accept illness as inevitable. This blend of experience—the present and past mixed in an infinite variety of ways—adds to the challenge of interviewing older patients.

This chapter deals with the process of interviewing the aged, unique aspects of the content of such interviews, and some of the common problems encountered.

2 THE PROCESS OF THE INTERVIEW

With older patients, the physical setting may be a decisive factor in making an interview effective. Adequate lighting is particularly important since many older patients have reduced visual acuity. The light should clearly illuminate the interviewer's face, so that lip reading can be accomplished. Because many elderly persons (45-50 percent) have decreased auditory acuity as well,[4] speaking clearly and distinctly is appreciated. The volume of one's voice should be raised only if necessary. Some older persons may be offended if the voice is raised without need.

It is extremely important that the clinician introduce himself initially. Other people were raised in a time when propriety and decorum were held in greater respect. Furthermore, many older persons harbor apprehensions about the medical profession. A measure of politeness helps to set them at ease. Most older people prefer to be addressed by their surnames rather than first names.

If the patient wears dentures, they should be in place. Embarrassment is a definite deterrent to open communication. Com-

munication of certain words is more difficult with the dentures out
and recognition of facial, non-verbal cues may be affected as well.

Once these measures have been taken, the interviewer can proceed. As with other patients, one should begin with open-ended
questions. Most older patients will be able to respond to this type
of questioning without difficulty, and in these cases techniques
used do not differ significantly from those discussed in Chapter 2.
Some elderly patients, however, may not respond to open-ended
questions. It then becomes important to discern the reason for
their difficulty.

Many elderly patients are frightened when being interviewed by
a health professional. They may have fears of institutionalization
or hospitalization. They may have some difficulty with memory,
and the anticipation of an embarrassing discovery of their memory
loss may inhibit their ability to communicate. If a patient is un-
responsive, whatever the reason, it is wise to shift one's attention
to the process rather than attempting to convince the patient of
the need to answer one's questions.

> An eighty-five-year-old woman was being interviewed by a second-
> year medical student. The student began the interview by asking,
> "What sort of problems are you having?" The patient responded
> angrily, "You're the doctor; you tell me." The student answered,
> "You sound upset." The patient then admitted, "Well, wouldn't
> you be if your daughter just told you that it might be time to go into
> a nursing home?"

Many older patients have been in medical settings numerous
times. They are "experienced" patients and have often been
"trained" to give their history in response to a short question-and-
answer format. These patients may be uneasy with an open-ended
line of inquiry.

Some older patients have difficulty responding to questions that
pertain to feelings or psychological issues. Many were raised in a
social climate in which "personal" problems were not discussed,
sometimes not even in one's own family. They may also be less
likely to open up early in the interview, waiting instead until they

can feel a measure of trust in the interviewer. If reassurance or a gentle confrontation that this line of questioning appears to be difficult for the patient does not restore the flow of communication, it is best to summarize and move on.

> CLINICIAN: So you lost your husband twelve years ago. What was that like for you?
>
> PATIENT: I don't like to talk about it actually. (*Silence*)
>
> CLINICIAN: (*After a short silence*) This subject seems hard for you to talk about.
>
> PATIENT: Well, it sort of brings up bad memories.
>
> CLINICIAN: Bad memories?
>
> PATIENT: Yes. But what about my heart? Am I going to have to take that new medicine?
>
> CLINICIAN: Well, when you care to talk about it, I really would like to hear about the death of your husband. As to your medicine . . .

A common fear on the part of some clinicians is that the older patient will go off on a tangent and begin telling old stories. This common habit of the elderly to "reminisce" serves a variety of purposes. The primary one is to reintegrate the vast amount of previous experiences into the present. In that sense, reminiscing has a distinctly positive function. Some studies have shown that this type of reminiscence is associated with prevention of cognitive decline and memory loss.[5] However, it may also be evidence of some intellectual impairment, particularly if excessive. Patients with memory problems will "reminisce" because they cannot converse in the here-and-now. Such reminiscing is usually tangential, that is, it is not associated with the discussion at hand. A simple question such as, "And how does that relate to what we were discussing?" may get the patient back on track. The clinician must decide whether or not to interrupt the patient, based upon the estimated value of the patient's reminiscence and the time available to the clinician.

The timing involved in the use of questions is referred to as tempo, and the interviewing tempo is different with older patients. As a population, older patients do not generally show a noticeable decline in intellectual functioning with age.[6] However, the speed of responses to both non-verbal tasks and verbal questions does decline slightly with age. Older patients are less likely to take risks and less willing to make errors than younger patients.[7] Hence, they may "cogitate" over a question before answering. They also may not have the physical stamina for a long and detailed interview. Especially those who are frail may appreciate a suggestion that the interview be completed on a second visit.

Most older people depend upon their family for some degree of support. Therefore, it is important to consider whether a family member should also be interviewed when seeing the older patient. If any indication of memory problems is noted during the interview, then it is imperative to corroborate the information presented by the patient. In our society, it is usually daughters or daughters-in-law who are the primary care-givers to older relatives. These care-givers may provide quite a different picture than that presented by the patient.

> During the interview, a seventy-five-year-old man gladly described his daily activities: working in his garden, going for a walk with his dog in the afternoon, and reading extensively. When the daughter was interviewed later, she reported that although he had had a large garden in the past, he had been housebound for the last three years and only left home for visits to the doctor.

Friends play an important role in the maintenance of social skills and in providing care to some patients. They will often accompany the patient to a hospital or office in times of distress. These friends may likewise be included in an interview after the first private one. They can corroborate details, such as the patient's activities or dates or problems, and can give the clinician an opportunity to witness the patient's style of communication with others.

In summary, though the process of interviewing older adults is usually very similar to that of interviewing younger patients, certain adjustments must often be made. Paying attention to the presence of sensory organ deficits associated with aging permits two-way communication. Allowing the patient to reminisce may help the older person integrate past experiences into the present. The timing of questions, and allowing for slower response time, will decrease both the patient's and the clinician's frustration. Finally, viewing the patient as a member of a family or other support system helps the interviewer understand the patient as a whole person.

3   THE CONTENT OF THE INTERVIEW

There are a few major differences in content between interviews of younger and older patients. One of the main differences is the large role that social-support systems play in maintaining health and in coping with disease. Although elderly persons suffer multiple medical problems, those who do not have a strong support system, either family or friends, are likely to do less well when ill. They utilize social services to a greater extent and are more likely to become residents of long-term care institutions.[8] Furthermore, their dependence on social-support systems is largely influenced by their ability to care for themselves. The elderly person's daily activities, his ability to perform self-care skills, and social-support systems are collectively called the "patient profile."

Patient Profile

As we grow older, variability of physiologic function from individual to individual increases. There is also more variability in the activities of daily living—those functions that one must perform in order to live independently. Dressing, toileting, preparing and consuming food, and ambulation are taken for granted by most younger people. Limitations in any of these areas can be a severe deterrent to independence, and such limitations occur more frequently as people age. These activities are best measured by asking patients to describe the last few meals prepared, watching them remove a sweater or shirt before the physical exam, and observing them as they get out of a chair or walk down the hall. Any activity that has been reported by the patient but not observed by the interviewer may need to be substantiated by other family members if the clinician has reason to doubt the patient's account.

The older person should be questioned about involvement in church groups, senior citizen centers, day care centers, or other social activities. Hobbies can be a positive factor in adjusting to retirement. Pets tend to increase an older person's sense of responsibility and companionship.[9]

Because many elderly persons survive on fixed incomes, knowledge of the person's living arrangements is helpful. Does the area have a high crime rate? Is the house safe as far as locks and exits are concerned? What is the patient's income? Obviously, those living on Social Security may have difficulty following a health professional's recommendations if the costs are too high.

Two areas often neglected when interviewing an older person are sex and the use of alcohol. Contrary to popular belief, most men continue to be sexually active into their seventh or even eighth decades.[10] Although older women maintain sexual activity less frequently, this probably has more to do with lack of partners (women outnumber men almost two to one after the age of seventy-five) than lack of interest. Indeed, over 65 per cent of those over sixty-five expressed interest in sexual activities when interviewed.[11] While it may not be mentioned in the first interview, sex should be discussed as the doctor-patient relationship develops.

The elderly are at high risk for developing alcoholism and one can expect one in ten to be alcoholic.[12] They have a higher rate of illness, poverty, and depression than the general population. Many suffer from loneliness, a common source of much problem drinking. Perhaps it is difficult for some interviewers to conceive of a seventy-five-year-old woman who reminds them of their grandmother being an alcoholic. Reticence in asking about alcohol intake is understandable but must be overcome if a complete history is to be taken.

Past Medical History

The past medical history of an older person can be quite extensive. Multiple medical problems and numerous past operations are not an uncommon pattern. How can all this information be managed? An emphasis on how any problem in the past may affect the patient's present-day functioning will help to keep the past medical information in perspective. For instance, except for rheumatic fever, childhood illnesses are unlikely to affect the older patient at the present time. However, in the patient with a recent stroke the past history of high blood pressure or diabetes is likely to be of extreme importance. The patient's present problem should lead the clinician in his or her pursuit of the past history.

A form, completed by the patient, containing a checklist of past medical and surgical problems will help to save time and allow more attention to be given to the patient during the interview. Having the patient bring old medical records from previous physicians provides details regarding past diagnoses and medications used as well as previously performed diagnostic tests.

Mental Status Examination

Only 5 per cent of the population over the age of sixty-five suffers from dementia or cognitive impairment.[13] However, approximately 20 per cent of those over eighty have this disorder, which was formerly called "senility." Patients with this problem are well represented in health care settings. Surprisingly, it is not uncommon to fail to recognize that one is interviewing a patient with dementia. This is so because personality and intelligence are two separate functions. A person's personality forms very early in life and is unlikely to be affected by the early stages of dementia. He or she may be affable and able to carry on a conversation without apparent difficulty. It is only when the patient's memory is actually tested that the cognitive impairment is discovered.

A seventy-nine-year-old woman was interviewed by a nurse practitioner in a geriatric clinic. The patient described her home in honest terms, saying that since her husband had died she really didn't keep her house as clean as she used to. However, she preferred to spend her time gardening and reported raising three varieties of orchids. She spoke freely and did not exhibit any unusual uneasiness during the

interview. However, upon specific questioning, she was unsure about
the date and could not remember her address or her age.

The mental status exam adds objective measurements of cognitive function to the subjective data gleaned during the interview.
The Short Portable Mental Status Questionnaire has been used
extensively in geriatric populations and is well validated.[14] It can
be given in about ten minutes and can be repeated over time to
assess changes in cognitive function.

It is important to put the patient at ease before administering
the test. For this reason it should usually be given at the end of
the interview. It is best introduced as "another method of evaluating your health, like the physical exam." The interviewer may
wish to add, "Although some of these questions may seem simple
and others difficult, they will help me to select the best treatment." If the patient shows some exasperation with failure during
the test, he should be encouraged to continue after a supportive
comment about the difficulty.

Some patients may attempt to explain away their difficulty in
recalling the date or the name of a president. Common responses
include, "Oh, my eyesight is pretty bad, so I never look at the
paper," or "The president? Why bother, they're all crooks anyway." Encouragement to try to answer will help the clinician
separate patients with severe cognitive disabilities (e.g., one who
says June 6, 1945, instead of December 3, 1984) from depressed
patients, who have difficulty answering but, with support, can
accurately name the date.

Should the patient make mistakes during the mental status
exam, it is important to recognize them and provide the correct
answers. Demented patients often know that they have a problem
with memory, and by recognizing the difficulty the clinician can
help reorient the patient. This, of course, should be said in a caring
and non-judgmental way.

Family History

The family history, like the past medical history, can be extensive
with older patients. The use of a family genogram—drawn with

the patient observing—often helps in obtaining information in the shortest amount of time. The symbols can be explained to the patient as the figure develops. Interestingly, information regarding family interactions is often volunteered when this method is used.

> An older man had finished describing his main problems. While the physician was diagraming his family, the patient admitted to having a brother whom he had not mentioned previously. His brother had died of a heart attack two years before. The patient expressed the fear that his own high blood pressure might also lead to a heart attack. When asked how he dealt with his brother's death, he said, "Oh, I just put it out of my mind."

A family genogram will also provide a more accurate picture of marriage relationships and present support systems. It can serve as a method for both obtaining and recording a large amount of information, negating the need for a lengthy narrative account of the patient's family history.

Medications

Approximately 85 per cent of the elderly are on at least one prescription drug.[15] The number regularly taking at least one over-the-counter drug is even higher.[16] While some of these drugs are relatively innocuous, the risk of overmedication and adverse drug reactions is greatly magnified by multiple use. Thus, it is essential to ascertain all the patient's present medications (and as many of the past ones as can be remembered).

Nutrition

The elderly represent the age group that runs the highest risk of malnutrition in our society. Inadequate income, physical difficulties in preparing meals and shopping, inadequate knowledge of the nutritional shortcomings of high-carbohydrate "fast foods," and individual taste preferences all contribute to malnutrition. The patient should be queried as to what he ate *that day* as a sample of daily intake. Asking how foods are bought and prepared may illuminate problems. Inquiries should be made into the use of home-delivered meal programs, such as Meals on Wheels, or of food stamps.

Exercise

An oft-used phrase in the care of the older person is, "Use it or lose it." This admonition applies to a great number of bodily functions, such as muscle strength, gait stability, and cardiovascular reserve. It also applies to cognitive functioning. Not only is exercise a vital way of maintaining functions, but cessation of heretofore regular exercise can be a sign of physical illness or depression.

Regular exercise can take many forms in older people. Gardening, woodworking, lawn care, walking, and calisthenics are common. These methods of maintaining physical function should be reinforced as a positive method of health promotion.

4 PROBLEMS IN INTERVIEWING OLDER ADULTS

There are several common difficulties in interviewing older patients. Some are a result of normal physiologic changes associated with aging, while others are due to the illnesses themselves. Both types of problems will be discussed in this section.

Some older persons have a multitude of chronic health problems. The interplay between these problems is complex and often unpredictable. Hence, the chief complaint is likely to be less decisive than with younger patients. The patient may first present a long-standing problem, one felt to be most important by the patient's children, or even one that the patient feels may be most interesting to the doctor. By asking the patient, "Which problem is most strongly interfering with your life right now?" one can help determine a path of diagnosis and treatment.

As people get older, they often speak of health problems in nonspecific terms. This phenomenon has several causes. Normal changes resulting from aging, such as decreased pain sensation, decreased nerve conduction velocity, and decreased temperature responses, can contribute to an altered reporting of illness. In addition, many of the afflictions experienced by an older person may be mistakenly perceived as a normal part of aging. Loss of hearing, poor vision, shortness of breath, decreased exercise tolerance, sexual dysfunction, and even incontinence, though treatable, may be perceived by the patient as just another part of "getting old." Unfortunately because they are subject to the same myths about old age, clinicians may contribute to this attitude.

A seventy-year-old widowed man reported to his physician that he had been impotent for the last six months. This was particularly distressing because impotence had rarely occurred before in his life and he had recently developed a relationship with a new companion. He was contemplating marriage but was frightened due to his change of sexual function. When he told his physician of these problems, the doctor said, "Well, we all have to get old some day." The patient was later seen by a different physician, who changed his anti-hypertensive medications, and the problem was resolved.

Many of the problems troubling older patients may, in fact, be non-specific. The most common of these include: "slowing down," either physically or mentally; weakness or tiredness; dizziness or falling; "rheumatism," which the patient may experience not only as joint pain but even as bone pain; anorexia or weight loss; and decreased libido. These problems may have their genesis in a remediable cause and deserve investigation.

Some elderly patients may be reticent about discussing their problems openly. They may appear suspicious or even paranoid. Some insight into this behavior can be gained from studies indicating that among the greatest fears of older persons is that of being "put away" or institutionalized.[17] In the patient's mind, it is a representative of the health care system—a doctor, social worker, or nurse—who is most likely to initiate placement in a long-term care setting. A clear statement to the patient that the goal of an intervention is to extend or ensure the patient's capacity to live independently (if that is indeed the case) may help to allay this fear.

Finally, there is another aspect of the presentation of illness that tends to distinguish older from younger patients, namely, physical illness that presents itself as psychological problems or vice versa. This phenomenon is different from a psychosomatic disorder. In the elderly, the person with an organic illness may have no physical complaints. The person with a severe psychological problem (e.g., depression) may have no psychological symptoms, instead complaining of multiple aches and pains. A major depression may precede by as much as six months the diagnosis of cancer. Certain endocrine problems, such as hypothyroidism, may present itself as depression or psychosis. Furthermore, the diagnosis of depression can be difficult. Even a severely depressed patient may not report feelings of hopelessness or loss of libido. Only the common signs of depression, such as early-morning wakening or change in appetite, may be mentioned. Because the older person was brought up at a time when feelings were not expressed as readily, especially to strangers, they may refrain from admitting to depression during the interview. Instead, they may present multiple physical complaints with little evidence of a depressed mood.

There are a number of approaches to this difficult problem. A new, serious decline in an older person's health or functioning should never be ascribed to "getting old" without adequately investigating the possibility of covert problems. An accurate history of the decline, a complete physical exam, and appropriate diagnostic tests will usually uncover hidden illnesses that are being expressed as psychological symptoms. Occasionally an older person will require a trial of anti-depressant medication after such an evaluation. But take heart—even the most experienced clinician may have difficulty distinguishing depression from organic illness in older patients.

5   CONCLUSION

This chapter has presented some of the special considerations one must take into account when interviewing an older patient. Certain aspects of the process of the interview, such as paying attention to sensory deficits and the importance of reminiscence, were discussed. The content of the history may also differ from that of a younger person. The wide variety of backgrounds and experiences and the diversity of medical problems require from the clinician a blend of practiced interviewing skills and a warm, empathetic approach. To paraphrase Sir William Osler, it is not enough to know what kind of disease the patient has but what kind of patient has the disease.

REFERENCES

1. Facts About Older Americans, 1979. U.S. Department of Health and Human Services, Office of Human Development Services, Administration on Aging, HHS Publication No. 80-20006, 1980.
2. Fact Book on Aging, Research and Evaluation Department, National Council on Aging, Washington, D.C., 1978.
3. La Rue, A., L. Bank, L. Jarvik, and M. Hetland, "Health in Old Age: How Do Physicians' Ratings and Self-ratings Compare?" *Journal of Gerontology*, 34:687-691, 1979.
4. Von Leden, H., "Speech and Hearing Problems in the Geriatric Patient," *Journal of the American Geriatric Society*, 25:422-426, 1977.
5. Butler, R. N., "The Life Review: An Interpretation of Reminiscence in the Aged, *Psychiatry*, 26:65-76, 1963.
6. Willis, S. L., and P. B. Battes, "Intelligence in Adulthood and Aging: Contemporary Issues," in L. W. Poon (ed.), *Aging in the 80's*. Washington, D.C.: American Psychological Association, 1980, pp. 260-272.
7. Heyn, J. E., J. R. Barry, and R. H. Pollack, Problem-solving as a Function of Age, Sex, and the Role Appropriateness of the Problem Content," *Experimental Aging Research*, 4:505-519, 1978.
8. Kane, R. L., and R. A. Kane, "Care of the Aged: Old Problems in Need of New Solutions," *Science*, 200:913-919, 1978.
9. Butler, R. N., and M. I. Lewis, *Aging and Mental Health*. St. Louis: Mosby, 1977, pp. 223-224.
10. McCarthy, P. "Geriatric Sexuality: Capacity, Interest and opportunity," *Journal of Gerontological Nursing*, 5:20-24, 1979.
11. Pfeiffer, E., and G. Davis, "Determinants of Sexual Behavior in the Elderly," *Journal of the American Geriatric Society*, 20:151-158, 1972.

12. Wattis, J. D. "Alcohol Problems in the Elderly," *Journal of the American Geriatric Society*, 29:131-134, 1981.
13. A Chartbook of the Federal Council on Aging. U.S. Department of Health and Human Services, Office of Human Development Services, Administration on Aging, HHS Publication No. 81-20704, 1981, p. 33.
14. Pfeiffer, E. "A Short Portable Mental Status Questionnaire for the Assessment of Organic Brain Deficit in Elderly Patients," *Journal of the Geriatric Society*, 23:433-441, 1975.
15. Law, R., and C. Chalmers, "Medicines and Elderly People: A General Practice Survey," *British Medical Journal*, 1:565, 1976.
16. Kiernan, P. J., and J. B. Isaacs, "Use of Drugs by the Elderly," *Journal of the Royal Society of Medicine*, 74:196, 1981.
17. Butler, R. N., and M. I. Lewis, *Common Emotional Problems in Aging and Mental Health*. St. Louis: Mosby, 1977, pp. 34-51.

8

INTERVIEWING THE FAMILY

Families play an important role in the onset of and recovery from illness. Illness frequently occurs at times of family crisis. Family members often call the clinician for explanations, advice, or reassurance. All clinicians need effective family interviewing skills to provide care that is comprehensive and compassionate.

TYPES OF FAMILIES

The most common type of family in the United States is the nuclear family, comprised of a father, mother, and often children. The nuclear family usually lives separate from, though sometimes close to, at least one set of grandparents. The nuclear family may be greatly affected by an illness among one of its members, particularly if the hospitalized patient is the mother of small children.[1]

Some families, more commonly those from minority groups and immigrant families, include other relatives such as grandparents and cousins. These are called extended families. They may consist of members of three generations living in one household. There are a number of advantages to a larger extended family, such as increased income and shared child care, but there may also be additional stresses. Examples are competition for attention among family members and blurring of lines of authority. Extended families may be closely knit and the illness of any member will usually have an impact on all the others.

Finally, there are alternatives to these more traditional models. Single-parent families are growing in number with the rise in divorce rates. Gay or lesbian couples may also have children from previous marriages or as a result of adoption. The adoption of children by unmarried members of religious orders is perhaps the newest type of alternative family. Each of these types has its own specific set of stresses and is likely to need the attention of a health care worker at some time.

THE CONCEPT OF FAMILY ILLNESS

Although most health care workers tend to view the patient as an isolated entity, the patient usually views himself as a member of a family. Both the patient and the family must cope with a serious change in that person's health status.[2] How the family will cope with an illness among one of its members can be looked at from a systems point of view.

A systems approach proposes that the individual patient is a "symptom carrier whose behavior, thoughts, physical state, and response to illness are influenced as much by the family with whom he/she lives as the disease process with which he/she is burdened."[3] An example of such a symptom carrier is the child with a behavioral problem in school. Traditionally the child is viewed as having a problem in need of correction. However, a family interview might uncover the fact that this child is afraid to leave his mother at home alone because she is an alcoholic who falls frequently. His "behavioral problems" have allowed him to stay at home to care for his mother. He is thus the "identified patient" in this family system, but not the one who is most ill.

Families tend to go through a predictable set of experiences when one member develops a serious illness. This normal process has been described as the "Illness Trajectory" by Burr and Good.[4]

The first phase of the Illness Trajectory is the "Onset of Illness Phase." It usually takes place before the diagnosis of a "disease."

If the illness is developing slowly, family members may notice changes in the patient's behavior or activities that cause concern. Depending on the family's communication style, these concerns may be discussed promptly or may remain unspoken, which then causes increased anxiety. In the case of a sudden heart attack, this phase will be quite rapid. With many illnesses (such as emphysema) it will be more gradual and may often be filled with uncertainty. Family members may seek the advice of clinicians during this time about a "change" in the family member with whom they are concerned. They may also label the patient a "complainer" because the disease may not be advanced enough to cause outright "illness," just a change in the patient's physical or emotional responses. However, as the problem progresses the diagnosis usually becomes clear.

The second phase is the "Impact Phase." The moment of being told the diagnosis is often remembered by the patient as the most difficult time in the course of an illness. This is particularly the case when the patient becomes depressed or withdrawn and when the family tries to cope with the patient's response through denial. How the patient adjusts to the illness will be greatly influenced by the way in which the family responds. Some families encourage open discussion of feelings and plans for dealing with the illness. These families may actually become stronger as a result of the illness. Others, usually those families that were having difficulties before the illness, will have even more trouble when a family member becomes ill. The additional strain on family communication may upset a delicate balance and have a disruptive effect.

The "Therapeutic Phase" then follows. While the patient is receiving medical attention, it is important to observe which family member assumes responsibility and to maintain good communication with that person. The hospitalization of different family members will have a different impact on the family. When mothers are hospitalized, there is a high risk of family disorganization, creating discomfort for all. When children are hospitalized, the child may experience feelings of abandonment, while parents may feel guilty over not having "protected" their youngster from illness. Though usually irrational, these feelings affect the way the family copes with the illness and with other stresses that may impinge on it. It will certainly affect their relations with health care professionals involved in the care of the patient.

As the disease is being treated, the family goes through the "Early Recovery Phase." Here the family may experience an unanticipated "letdown," a delayed reaction to the stress of the illness. During this time the clinician may find that the patient appears to cling to his illness. This is particularly true of children. The patient attempts to prolong the positive feelings and responses one gets when ill and being cared for. This often occurs in families that were in a state of discord (such as that resulting from marital problems) before the child became ill. The parents may be so involved in the care of the child that they temporarily put aside their differences and argue less. The child may then more or less unconsciously wish to remain ill to keep the parents together.

Finally, as the patient recovers or adapts to a chronic disease, there is the "Adjustment to Permanency of Outcome Phase." The clinician must continue to be aware that unwillingness to face (not necessarily "accept") the reality of the illness may be a sign of family discord. In this case, as well as during the Impact Phase and Early Recovery Phase, family conferences may be extremely important in resolving the difficulties. Awareness of these phases of the family's experience in illness will help the clinician provide preventive counseling and advice.

Family Dynamics

Every family has its unique communication style, rules, alliances, belief systems, and ways of reducing tension. While families can provide much support to one of its members during an illness, they may also play a part in its causation. Illness may cause great instability in one family, whereas in another family a similar illness can help stabilize a family in discord.

Mr. I suddenly developed epilepsy at age fifty-nine. A CT scan of the brain revealed a tumor. All his life he had been a computer expert who maintained "control" over his family. His disease forced his wife to assume many of the household financial decisions, a job with which she was quite unaccustomed. Shortly thereafter she suffered a heart attack, having had no predisposing symptoms. Their daughter, a banker, then assumed responsibility for their financial affairs.

A common family "rule," often seen in middle-class families, is that one doesn't talk about family problems to "strangers." Strangers may include health professionals. In one respect, all rules may serve to maintain the family's equilibrium. Equilibrium, or homeostasis, refers to the ability of the family to continue functioning even under difficult conditions. In that regard, it isn't a question of maintaining the status quo but of making a constant set of adjustments to help the family meet the needs of its members. Hence, the principal of homeostasis may also be applied to a family in disharmony.

As a result of family rules limiting communication with outsiders, or as a way of maintaining equilibrium, some but not all of the family members may form alliances with others. Permanent alliances are often a sign of family discord and may decrease the family's ability to cope with problems.

Occasionally a particular member is blamed for all of the problems encountered by the family. Such "scapegoating" is another sign of family discord. Though scapegoating may provide the first step in maintaining equilibrium, it leads to later problems which may become serious. Strict authoritarian families run the highest risk for scapegoating. Because children are often made the scapegoat, serious behavioral problems may be the outcome for the child.

It is important to remember that the patient being cared for may be the one person whose response to ongoing family problems is the development of symptoms. As mentioned earlier, this family member is called the "identified patient." Directing attention to that person's acute symptoms does not address the question of the source of the problem. In the case of the child with a behavioral problem, described earlier in this chapter, an interview with the whole family can make it clear that the child is only one member in a group of people with problems. Children with frequent infections or accidents are also prone to be the "identified patient" in a family in discord.[5, 6] While observations of the various roles played in the family system may be helpful to the clinician, referral to a person skilled in family therapy is usually necessary in this case.

The Family Life Cycle

There are many opportunities to interview families other than in disease-related circumstances. Families go through a more or less regular series of changes, each associated with specific stresses.[7] Members of the family may seek out health care workers at those times for advice or counsel. In these cases family interviewing can be used as a health maintenance tool. "Anticipatory guidance" can be given as to the kinds of stresses one might experience, or simple reassurance that their concerns are normal. The family life cycle includes:

STAGE	STRESSES
Forming the family	New living situation Adjusting to partner's desires Adjusting to partner's family Finances
Birth of first child	Changes in mother's work patterns Child-rearing Finances
Children in school	School performance Behavioral problems
Children leave home	Re-defining parental roles Second career/mother's working

Retirement	Re-defining self-worth
	More time together
	Adjusting to health problems
	Finances
Death	Adapting to widowhood
	Finances

Because divorce occurs so frequently, it might be considered an alternate phase of the family life cycle. Family members may visit physicians more frequently around the time of divorce.

SITES FOR FAMILY INTERVIEWS

Most clinicians are probably used to the hospital as the main site for family interviews. Indeed, discussions with the patient's family is a crucial part of medical care. Opportunities for such discussions abound. Key times when family discussions would be most helpful include:

1. Diagnostic phase—particularly in the case of the very young or very old, where corroboration of information is needed.
2. Explaining the diagnosis—especially with life-threatening illnesses such as heart attacks, cancer, or chronic illness such as spinal cord injuries, where family involvement will be needed.
3. Discussing treatment options—adherence to medication regimens has been shown to be enhanced when family members are involved. When the treatment entails ongoing discomfort for the patient (e.g., surgery, special diets, or chemotherapy), a family conference is particularly helpful.[8, 9, 10]
4. Pre-discharge planning—summarizing all the findings, treatments, and recommendations for follow-up helps the patient and family carry through with medical plans.

There are some drawbacks to the hospital as an interview site. The patient and family are on the health care worker's "turf" and may feel inhibited about disclosing information or expressing concerns. It is often difficult to convene many family members at the time of traditional rounds in the morning. Clinicians interested in family interviews may need to schedule special afternoon or early-evening sessions. Children may be excluded unnecessarily by bureaucratic visiting rules.

The office or clinic as a site for the family interview may make it possible to obtain information that could not have been gained in a hospital setting. For one thing, the patient is usually dressed in street clothes, providing him with some extra measure of confidence. The time of day set aside for an interview in an office is less restricted and children can more easily be included.

Should the patient reside in a nursing home, a family conference can be held at the patient's bedside or in a larger meeting room. Institutionalized patients may feel very lonely. A family interview affords them attention and allows the clinician the opportunity to see the patient's family "in action," as well as to gain useful historical information.

Finally, the patient's home should not be forgotten as an excellent site for family interviews. Here the patient and the family are on their own turf. It is the clinician who is the guest. The most accurate picture of family interaction is seen in the home. At home people tend to regress. One can then observe the patient's level of dependency on family members. The family's capacity to provide care can be observed. Direct suggestions can often be made. The home is the ideal place for a family interview.

THE FAMILY INTERVIEW IN MEDICAL CARE

Acute Health Crises

The patient with a newly diagnoses serious illness offers an excellent opportunity for a family interview. The best times for such an interview are shortly after the diagnosis has been made and sometime before discharge from the hospital. This allows the patient enough time to be free of the effects of anesthetic agents or simply to let the diagnosis "sink in." It also allows adequate time before the patient goes home to answer questions and make plans for the future. Patients with heart attacks, strokes, or cancer should certainly be given this opportunity. Most families are quite willing to adjust their schedules to meet the needs of the clinician if enough advance warning is given. Other, less serious problems can also be addressed through a family interview. Any discussion of sexual problems should include the patient's partner at the interview as often as possible. Behavioral problems in children can usually only be resolved with adequate family involvement.

The death of any family member, particularly that of a child, creates the greatest stress for a family. Deaths that occur in hospitals are particularly stressful. The incidence of illness among the survivors is more frequent than if the death occurred at home.[11, 12, 13] Some of the stress can be alleviated by a series of family interviews in which the survivor's responses can be expressed and given support. Questions can be answered. The grieving process is facilitated by ongoing discussions and through the expression of emotions. The passage of time is, of course, most helpful.

Finally, the diagnosis of an inherited disorder (such as sickle-cell anemia or Tay-Sachs disease) provides yet another chance to interview families as a whole. Obtaining an accurate genetic history is only one goal of this meeting. The family's emotional responses and concerns about future pregnancies should also be discussed. This setting provides ample opportunity to go beyond childbirth planning. Options for later treatment can be discussed as well.

Health Care in Chronic Illness

All chronic diseases can be difficult experiences for patients and their families. Because changes in the health status of a person with a chronic illness are less obvious than in acute illness, the need for family interviews may be underestimated. There are, however, suitable circumstances where a family conference can be useful. The patient not responding to therapy may be having difficulty in complying with the treatment regimen. Compliance has been shown to be enhanced with more family involvement. When the family is providing the care at home, as in severe emphysema or in neurologic problems, there are often many questions best addressed in family settings. When the family is anticipating institutionalization of an older person, a family meeting is essential. It provides an opportunity to more accurately assess the need for such a change as well as to deal with the guilt feelings so commonly experienced by family members.

When discussing a patient's desire for further interventions, such as cardiopulmonary resuscitation, "living wills," or a request for more vigorous or heroic therapies, such as chemotherapy for advanced cancer, the involvement of family members helps the patient feel less alone and fearful. From a medico-legal standpoint, such decisions are less risky if the family is involved.

Diagnostic and Treatment Dilemmas

An important instance in which family meetings are most helpful is the patient who represents a diagnostic or treatment dilemma. The patient whose "tests are all normal," or who has persistently asked many doctors, "Why can't any of you find the problem?" often has a family problem that is being masked by the illness.

> A fifty-eight-year-old woman complained of constant left facial pain of seven years' duration. Complete work-ups, including special x-rays, revealed no cause. Relaxation/meditation, acupuncture, electrical stimulation, and drugs all gave no relief.
>
> Upon interviewing the family, it became apparent that the patient was dissatisfied with her husband, aged eighty-five years. Her only satisfaction came when one or both of her adult daughters came over to take her to one of her many doctors' appointments.

In such a case, further diagnostic studies using the most advanced technology would only lead to greater expense and the inevitable question, "Why can't you doctors find the problem?" The problem was discovered in the course of a family interview, not by reading an x-ray.

> During the family interview the patient was instructed to communicate all her "medical worries" only to the physician, and not her daughters. The daughters were instructed to spend the same amount of time they had given to taking their mother to doctors' appointments to shopping or dining with her. The patient's pains gradually disappeared.

CONDUCTING A FAMILY INTERVIEW

Convening the Family Members

In hospital settings the family interview can be most easily convened by speaking with the patient about the need for such a meeting. Occasionally, as in the case of a comatose patient or a child, the spouse or parent will need to be contacted. It is important to have the patient's permission so as not to undermine the clinician-patient relationship. Once permission has been gained, it must be decided who would be the most appropriate person to contact other family members. Usually this contact can be made by the patient, but the "authority" of the physician can be used to gather the family together, particularly when the family is disengaged or very distraught as a result of the patient's illness.

In some larger families various members may contact health care workers individually. This is time-consuming and may lead to distortion of information learned secondhand. When this occurs, a remark by the clinician such as, "I've now spoken with several members of your family and would like to meet with all of you together to summarize the information we know so far and to give you an opportunity to ask any questions," will serve to set up the first interview.

In outpatient settings a time should be scheduled when the entire family can meet. While interesting family interviews can occur in a crowded examination room, it is preferable to have a meeting room with enough chairs for all family members. When the family is convened, it is important to observe the early inter-action of the various members. Where do they choose to sit? Does one person "take charge" at the meeting? How do parents manage children's activities and questions? Are there any obvious alliances among members? Perhaps most important, is there a "scapegoat" in the family for whom problems are blamed?

There are only rare instances when the patient should not be involved in the interview. Such a case might be a patient with severe communication difficulties (such as a stroke) who might not be able to follow the conversation, leading to increased anx-iety. Even in these cases, the clinician and family should meet with the patient afterward to share basic information discussed.

Opening the Interview

There are a number of ways to begin the family interview. The choice will depend upon the reason for the meeting. If the original purpose of a family meeting was to discuss diagnostic findings, that should be simply stated. If the goal of the session is to discuss treatment options, then more open-ended probing of the patient's and family members' feelings are in order. In general, it is impor-tant to begin interviews in an open-ended fashion because the clinician's concerns may not be the same as the family's.

Mrs. G. has recently had a computed tomography scan of the abdo-men that revealed massively enlarged lymph nodes. She has no peripheral nodes and feels reasonably well. Her physician has known her for some time and remembers she has a passionate fear of cancer.

DOCTOR: Mary has told me that she shared with you the results of her x-ray. What questions do you have?

This type of opening is neutral enough to allow a wide variety of questions, from clarification of the diagnosis (since the patient may not transmit that information accurately) to discussing the various treatment options. Family members may also ask questions about the cause of the illness or their role in ongoing care. Since the entire family is hearing the information together, there is less chance of misunderstanding.

It is often helpful to convene families not only to transmit diagnostic understanding but also to help them cope with the feelings that attend the diagnosis of a life-threatening disease.

> Mr. S. is recovering from a heart attack. He has often expressed how concerned he is about his family because they all seem to be treating him as if he were "fine china that would break if they touched me."
>
> NURSE: I asked you all to meet together because, in my experience, most families have a lot of questions about how they should treat their loved one after a heart attack. How about you?

Here the clinician helps the family discuss the problem openly and can dispel some of the common myths held by lay persons, such as the notion that all heart attack patients are fragile.

Some families have strong disagreements about treatment plans. A group interview serves to help families make decisions together about these difficult problems.

> Mrs. G. is contemplating not having a surgical procedure to diagnose the cause of her enlarged lymph nodes, as her doctor had advised. Her husband wants her to try faith healing. Her daughter thinks she ought to have the surgery.
>
> DOCTOR: Mrs. G. is facing a very difficult decision about whether or not to have surgery. What do each of you think about that?

Although the clinician may have very strong opinions about the best choice, patients often make their decisions based upon a variety of advisers' opinions, usually placing high value on their family members' thoughts. The above opening also gives the clinician an opportunity to see how the family solves problems. The process of problem-solving will allow the clinician to observe family roles and develop plans for later work with the family. Families that have difficulty reaching consensus about such problems may do so because of the stress of the situation. However, their difficulty may also be evidence of pre-existing family discord. In that case the health crisis may provide an opportunity to identify a family's need for therapy. Appropriate referrals can then be made.

Eliciting Information

The next stage of the interview is the elicitation of more information. With some families this is easily accomplished, particularly those that are accustomed to open exchanges of feelings and reactions. Such a family will need an interviewer who uses facilitation to encourage the more quiet members to participate.

> Mrs. P., a woman with multiple medical complaints, was asked to bring her family in to discuss the results of a comprehensive exam. Her husband and daughter attended the interview. After the clinician opened the interview, the daughter spent much time inquiring about details of the examination. The husband was essentially silent.
>
> NURSE: Mr. P., I've noticed you've been sort of quiet while the rest of your family has been doing most of the questioning. Do you have any questions?
>
> MR. P. (*angrily*): Yeah, I'd like to know when she's going to be well again so our life can get back to normal.

Another method of eliciting information is to comment on the process of communication in the interview.

> The S. family was actively discussing whether their grandmother should come home after a serious illness or go to a nursing home. The patient's daughter, who would be caring for the grandmother, brought up a number of concerns about the option of home care. The rest of the family dismissed her concerns with little or no discussion.
>
> INTERVIEWER: I've noticed that each time your mother brings up a concern about her mother coming home, the rest of you seem to dismiss it.

Some families have a difficult time having a true discussion of an issue. One person, often the father, may dominate the discussion. The interviewer's skill will be sorely tested. In such a situation, the best approach may be to guide the discussion away from the facts and call attention to the process of discussing them. Calling attention to the lack of participation by family members other than the controlling member may open up the discussion. This may also help the family learn to communicate in a more open way.

It is extremely important not to take sides with particular family members. This kind of alliance will destroy the other family members' trust in the clinician and limit his further effectiveness. Alliances often occur in families. They may form because of similarities in philosophy. More commonly, however, they enable those in the family with less power to carry greater weight in decision-making. When such a family is having a heated argument, one member of the group may ask the clinician to decide for them. It is best to avoid providing "the answer." It is hardly likely that an answer will be the right one for all the members of the family. This can only lead to further conflict. One approach to this situation is exemplified in the next example:

> Mr. P. had been hospitalized recently. Some of his children wanted him to stop driving because his reflexes were too slow. One daughter asked the physician to "tell him he can't drive anymore." His son then said that if he can't drive "he'll just die."
>
> DOCTOR: I can see that you disagree about your father's driving after he is discharged from the hospital. I suggest that we discuss this question with him. I think he should hear about your concern for his safety as well as his independence.

This kind of statement identifies the underlying emotional concerns of the two sides without taking sides. It also clarifies the role of the clinician as patient advocate. Finally, it helps the family to work out their own problems together.

CLARIFYING CONTENT

The facts surrounding any medical problems constitute but one area, referred to as "content" in the family interview. While these

facts are crucial to the patient and his family in terms of understanding the problem, other concerns that are not so directly related to the problem also affect their understanding. These concerns are more emotionally laden and are often hidden.

One such concern has to do with guilt about causation of the
illness or accident. This is particularly true with parents of young
children who have accidents or become ill. While some parents
may be open about their concerns regarding their role in the illness, many may not. Others may present a deluge of questions,
often repeating the same or similar ones. Some parents may appear
to be more distressed than would be expected given the degree of
the illness. Feelings of guilt about one's role in the development
of an illness are not limited to parents of children. For instance,
spouses of alcoholics often believe they could have prevented the
alcoholic from drinking. Whenever family members share their
love for one person, they are likely to feel some responsibility for
that individual's health.

Nurse G., after cleansing a young boy's badly bruised leg, the result
of a fall from a bicycle, noticed that the father, Mr. K., appeared
quite angry with his wife.

NURSE G.: Mr. K., you look sort of irritated.
MR. K.: Well, I've told my wife not to let Paul ride that bike. Now
look what's happened.
NURSE G.: Mrs. K., how do you feel about the accident?

This kind of response helps the family talk out the problem without taking sides. The nurse does not give reassurance too soon (by
saying, "Oh, no, accidents will happen"). Children's accidents
happen more frequently during times of family stress,[14] so the ensuing discussion may help to prevent further calamities.

Another important area in many family discussions is concern
about changes in the relationships within the family due to illness.
Worries over overdependence, the later need for care, the ability to
provide a livelihood, and financial matters may weigh heavily on
some family members' minds. After certain illnesses, such as heart

attacks or cancer, sexual partners will usually be concerned about future sexual activity. The clinician should encourage the patients and their families to discuss these questions, in a sense giving them permission to do so. Anxiety can be lessened by stating that these are common questions under the circumstances.

If the illness has resulted in a major change in the patient's functional capabilities, such as the ability to walk, communicate, or attend to such daily needs as dressing, feeding, or toileting, it is incumbent on the clinician to bring the family together to talk about the impact of that change on the family. One example of such an impact is the fact that 50 per cent of married patients who have suffered spinal cord injuries get divorced within two years of the injury. It is not only important to discuss how the family will adapt but also how they feel about the change. If there are strong negative feelings on the part of some family members, it is likely that care giver-related problems (such as poor quality of care or even abuse) may ensue.[15] There may be a need to discuss such concerns without the patient being present. Many such problems need only be discussed and brought out into the open to begin the process of resolution. Others may require modification of the home environment, such as hiring a care-giver, to lessen the burden on family members under stress. Open confrontation of such problems helps decrease the long-term pressures on the family.

SUMMARY

Because our society is composed of a system of "families"—families of origin, extended families, families of friends—many individuals are affected when one person becomes ill. The family can help the patient to recover from illness, but it may also prolong or even prevent recovery. By using family-interviewing skills, the clinician can help families cope with the emotional and intellectual burden created by illness. According to an old Chinese saying, "Crisis equals danger plus opportunity." In a health care crisis, the clinician and patient may have an opportunity to help a troubled family. The opportunity comes in helping the family see illness as a chance to improve their communication and develop a deeper sense of love.

REFERENCES

1. Burr, B., and B. Good, "The Impact of Illness on the Family," in R. Rabel (ed.), *Family Medicine*. New York: Springer-Verlag, 1978, p. 228.
2. Klein, R., A. Dean, and M. Bogdoroff, "The Impact of Illness upon the Spouse," *Journal of Chronic Diseases*, 20:241, 1978.
3. Bauman, M., and N. Grace, "Family Process and Family Practice," *Journal of Family Practice*, 4:1135, 1977.
4. Burr and Good, op. cit., pp. 223-231.
5. Rogers, J., "Recurrent Childhood Poisoning as a Family Problem," *Journal of Family Practice*, 13:337, 1981.
6. Whitehead, L., "Sex Differences in Children's Responses to Family Stress: A Re-evaluation," *Journal of Child Psychology and Psychiatry*, 20:247, 1979.
7. Duvall, E. (ed.), *Family Development*, 4th ed. Philadelphia: J. B. Lippincott Company, 1971.
8. Steiell, J., "Medical Condition, Adherence to Treatment Regimens and Family Functioning," *Archives of General Psychiatry*, 37:1025, 1980.
9. Oakes, T., "Family Expectations and Arthritis Patient Compliance to a Hand-resting Splint Program," *Journal of Chronic Diseases*, 22:757, 1970.
10. Schultz, S., "Compliance with Therapeutic Regimens in Pediatrics: A Review of Implications for Social Work Practice," *Social Work Health Care*, 5:267, 1980.
11. Rees, W., and S. Lutking, "Mortality of Bereavement," *British Medical Journal*, 1:113, 1967.
12. Parkes, C., and R. Brown, "Health after Bereavement: A Controlled Study of Young Boston Widows and Widowers," *Psychosomatic Medicine*, 34:449, 1972.
13. Parkes, C., B. Benjamin, and R. Fitzgerald, "Broken Heart: A Statistical Study of Increased Mortality among Widowers," *British Medical Journal*, 1:740, 1969.

14. Huygen, F., *Family Medicine: The Medical Life History of Families.* The Netherlands: Dekker and Van de Vegt, 1978.

15. Cantor, M., "Strain among Care-givers: A Study of Experience in the United States," *The Gerontologist,* 23:597, 1983.

9

INTERVIEWING IN DENTISTRY

"Going to the dentist" provokes fear in many people. Because of fear, some people do not seek dental care until forced to do so by pain, infection, bleeding gums, or anxious relatives and acquaintances. As a result of delay, patients lose teeth unnecessarily and endure pain and disfigurement. When patients must undergo stressful, unplanned emergency treatment, their fear is reinforced.

Patients who receive regular dental care may also suffer from fears. They may fear that the dentist will find something requiring treatment; they may fear the anesthetic needle or the drill, with its noise and vibration; they may even fear the individual dentist.

Many of these fears are intrinsic to the traditional nature of dental practice. Dentistry evolved as a surgical discipline with emphasis on the repair of decayed teeth, extraction of bad teeth, and the making of artificial teeth. The profession has attracted individuals with scientific interests who like to work with their hands; many are less skilled in dealing with people. As a result, practitioners have often paid too little attention to the human factors involved in treating patients while seeking technical perfection in their work. These attitudes, coupled with the psychological and pain sensitivities of the mouth, lead inevitably to the fears and anxieties experienced by patients undergoing dental treatment. The fearful patient may in turn produce emotional reactions in the dentist that can ultimately have a wide range of adverse personal and professional effects.

Dentists treat two kinds of disease. Dental caries, or tooth decay, destroy the substance of the teeth. Periodontal disease affects the gums and tooth socket bone; this leads to loosening and eventual loss of the teeth. As dentistry matured scientifically, the primary cause of these dental diseases, bacterial deposits on the teeth, was discovered. As a result, dentists have altered emphasis from the mechanical repair of dental lesions to helping people understand their dental problems and teaching them how to take personal action to prevent serious dental disease.

Preventive health care measures require significant cooperation by patients. The clinician asks the patient to prevent a problem by taking action, such as using proper tooth-brushing techniques or using dental floss, rather than waiting until a problem requiring treatment has occurred. This approach to dental care is based on a relationship between patient and dentist characterized by mutual understanding of the nature of dental diseases and their prevention. This understanding requires clear, effective communication between dentist and patient.

Should dental treatment be necessary, patients' fears are markedly reduced, or eliminated altogether, if the patient and the dentist share a high degree of trust. A good initial interview is an important part of effective dental practice. The early establishment of trust and communication between dentist and patient reduces patients' vague fears, alleviates their anxieties concerning pain and discomfort, and serves to motivate them to adopt preventive self-care habits.

The interviewing model described in Chapters 2 and 3 applies to dental practice, and this chapter is addressed to that application. It emphasizes interviewing new patients. Excerpts of interviews with patients are presented to illustrate typical problems.

1   THE NATURE OF DENTAL PRACTICE

The personality of the dentist may interfere with or facilitate the establishment of cooperative relationships with patients. The orientation of dentists is sometimes associated with personality characteristics, such as a need for order and predictability that approaches compulsiveness. In some dentists, a tendency to inflexibility can be a problem. Dentists share the characteristics of the doctor's role described in Chapter 2; they may be tempted to rely too heavily on their authority to make patients follow treatment recommendations and, in so doing, may fail to consider the patient's need for support and trust, as well as his desire for a role in making decisions. The surgical nature of most dental procedures reinforces this tendency by requiring the patient to be passive and compliant while the dentist is active. Obvious clinical problems may tempt the dentist to start treatment without sufficient information about the patient's general health, social and family background, and emotional status, which is, of course, an error. Such an approach treats the patient as a passive subject and does little to reduce anxiety and fear. Dentists may resort to drugs in order to more easily control a patient's behavior and suppress fear, which unfortunately induces further passivity. While convenient during a surgical procedure, passivity does not help in creating a feeling of responsibility for self-care.

Efforts to carry out highly technical procedures in the confined area of the mouth, while at the same time adhering to a rigid work schedule, can be extremely stressful to the clinician. Patients' "uncooperative behavior," such as gagging, fidgeting, or not opening the mouth fully, often a manifestation of their anxiety, puts additional stress on the dentist.

Many dental patients are unaware that they are suffering from chronic dental diseases. Pain does not usually occur until the disease is in an advanced stage. This adds to the difficulty of teaching prevention and self-care; frequently the disease is far advanced before treatment begins.

Dentists often err in lecturing patients about treatment and preventive measures, without inquiring about their current understanding of their needs. Such lectures, which offer no opportunity for patients to participate, usually fail to motivate them to adopt new health care behavior. Successful long-term management of dental caries and periodontal disease depends on the clinician's ability to counsel and motivate patients effectively.

2   INTERVIEWING DENTAL PATIENTS

Effective open-ended interviewing can do much to improve traditional dental practice. If the dentist gives the patient the opportunity to provide important information in his own words, the dentist can help reduce much of the stress, anxiety, and poor communication common to dental practice. By actively listening to the patient, the dentist departs from the active doctor/passive patient model and demonstrates that the individual seeking treatment has an important role in successful therapy.

The Interview Setting

The dentist should provide a relaxed and non-threatening environment for the interview. His private office serves as an ideal setting, since it is free of dental equipment and other features that emphasize technical aspects of the dentist's role. The dentist should conduct the interview while he and the patient are seated in similar comfortable chairs arranged in such a way as to encourage dialogue. Many professional offices feature an imposing desk, though communication suffers when a big desk separates the patient and the doctor. If a desk is present, chairs arranged to enable the doctor and patient to converse on the same side of the desk, or to be separated only by a desk corner, will enhance the interview.

As a second choice, the dental treatment room may be used for the interview. If the patient is in a dental chair, it should be in an upright position at the same eye level as the interviewer. Keep instruments and other equipment out of sight until the interview is concluded. Every effort should be made to provide an environment that encourages feelings of comfortable participation between patient and doctor.

The Use of Questionnaires in Dental Practice

The data needed to provide effective dental care include the new patient's past medical history and current health status, past dental history and current complaints, psychological status, and feelings concerning both preventive health care and dentistry in general.

Questionnaires are useful in dental practice because they provide a means of obtaining certain kinds of information rapidly. The typical questionnaire contains a series of questions requiring yes or no answers. By its very nature, it cannot provide much information about the patient's emotional status and personal concerns. The dentist should review the questionnaire and question the patient to make sure significant facts have not been omitted and to explore information recorded. By using the questionnaire as a supplement to a good interview, the dentist emphasizes early interaction with patients on a personal level. Person-to-person communication, rather than an impersonal checklist, serves as the patient's introduction to the dentist's care.

Conducting the Interview

The following sequence has proved successful in integrating an open-ended interview with the care of new dental patients. While waiting in the reception area for the appointment to begin, the patient completes a questionnaire. Name, address, age, and other relevant personal information, including financial responsibility, past medical history, past dental history, and oral hygiene practices, are the areas of inquiry. The dentist reviews the form briefly before meeting the patient.

The dentist and new patient meet in the reception room and walk together to the interview area in the dentist's private office. The doctor begins the interview with an open-ended question and proceeds as described in Chapter 2; he ends it with a specific review of the responses to the questionnaire.

A staff member then shows the patient into a treatment room and prepares him for the clinical examination. During this time, the dentist writes a summary of the findings from the interview.

This includes an assessment of the patient's psychological status, his attitudes toward dental care, and a description of the dental problem.

The interview and the dentist's written summary usually can be completed in approximately twenty minutes. Many initial interviews take less time when there are no major psychological problems or when the history of the dental problem is simple. Occasionally an interview may be prolonged by difficulties the patient presents, such as severe anxiety, specific dental phobias, a complex history, or hostility. Time is well spent in discovering these problems and dealing with them during the interview, as it gives the dentist information that can be used to prevent even greater losses of time later in treatment.

3 EXAMPLES OF DENTAL PATIENT INTERVIEWS

To illustrate the use of open-ended interviewing in dentistry, a series of examples drawn from dental practice is presented hare. A variety of cases has been selected to demonstrate new patient interviews, problems associated with difficult, anxious patients or patients with acute symptoms, and the integration of a review of a questionnaire with an interview.

A New Patient Interview

Patient 1. Mrs. L. is a thirty-nine-year-old married woman. She has experienced chronic soreness and bleeding in one area of her mouth. She has been seen recently by her family dentist, followed by a periodontist and an internist. The conflicting recommendations of these practitioners have confused and upset her. She desires to resolve these conflicts and obtain treatment for her problem. She now seeks another professional opinion.

> DOCTOR: You were saying you had a sad story for me.
> PATIENT: This will be my second examination by a periodontist. All my gum troubles have happened in the last six months, as far as I'm concerned. I've had my teeth cleaned on my regular six-month

schedule. Now I find out my bridges are loose, and that a back tooth is loose.

DOCTOR: You say the bridges are loose?

PATIENT: Okay, the back molar is loose; that's holding the bridge. The other bridge was loose, too, and my dentist took it out; I don't know why. He put a temporary in until I can get to a periodontist. He said it looks like I have gum disease. Of course I went to a periodontist. He said I might lose the tooth, or I might not. He looked at my mouth and said my whole mouth must be worked on because I have gum disease. This upsets me no end. I had my teeth straightened and my bridges put in three years ago. At that time, supposedly, my mouth was okay, and I was told I should have my teeth the rest of my life. I just can't imagine how my mouth could fall apart in just six months. I'm a diabetic but I'm controlled. I went to my internist and he said he is not convinced that the diabetes has caused this gum disease. He doesn't buy that story. In the meantime, here I sit. What do I do now? Obviously, I care about my teeth or I wouldn't have taken care of them as much as I have. I'm just really upset about it.

DOCTOR: You refer to the internist not buying the story. What story?

PATIENT: Because I've got diabetes, my mouth is going bad. This is the reason they're giving me. . . .

DOCTOR: Who are "they"?

PATIENT: My dentist and the other periodontist. That's probably water under the bridge, but it upset me. I don't know whether it was just a bad guess that all this dental work three years ago would save my teeth. They hoped the bridges would last maybe ten or fifteen years; instead they've lasted less than four. I don't know what the problem is.

DOCTOR: Did you have a chance to talk with the other periodontist about treatment?

PATIENT: Yes, and he said that my whole mouth would have to be worked on. There would be some surgery involved, but he thought he could save the teeth. My regular dentist told me last night, after he read the report Dr. ———— had sent him, that he said this tooth was hopelessly involved. He told my doctor one thing and told me another. He told me he thought he could save this tooth. Well, it's obvious that it's gone now. I'm sure it is. I don't know . . .

DOCTOR: How did you feel about that?

PATIENT: I'm upset. I think I was more upset when I found out about my mouth and gum disease than I was when I found out that I had diabetes. I felt that I was taking care of my mouth, that I was doing what I was supposed to be doing. In a matter of six months I don't see how my mouth could have gotten so bad. And, of course, they are using diabetes as the reason. I don't know, maybe it's true, but I'm not totally convinced. I just don't believe that. I don't want to go through surgery unless I have to. That's not easy if you are a diabetic. So this whole situation upsets me; to think I have to go through this mess!

DOCTOR: You sound pretty discouraged.

PATIENT: I'm very discouraged with dentistry in general.

Later in the interview the patient referred to some uncomfortable temporary fillings:

PATIENT: I'm not going to be able to chew on this side of my mouth this weekend. I don't know what I'm going to do.

DOCTOR: You can't chew on the temporaries?

PATIENT: No. I'm . . . well, I don't want to go into it, as upset as I am. Really, I liked my own teeth. I planned on having them. My husband feels exactly the opposite. He could care less. My problem doesn't affect him. We've got a thing going too: I want to save my teeth and I'm the one that's ending up with all the gum disease. He really doesn't care and gets along okay. I'm not really getting much sympathy at home. I don't blame him; he spent a thousand dollars on my teeth three years ago. I work at least fifteen or twenty minutes on my teeth every night. I don't know what I'm doing wrong. I can't imagine what more I can do. I'm wondering if they can even be saved now. I wonder if it's worth it to go through more treatment and maybe in three years my teeth will have to be pulled anyway.

DOCTOR: Yes, with what's happened I can understand how you feel.

PATIENT: And yet I dread the thought of having my teeth pulled now.

DOCTOR: Yes, you're not that old.

PATIENT: No, I'm thirty-nine years old. My family has a history of

having dentures early. I thought it was because they haven't taken
care of their teeth. I feel I've taken care of my teeth, yet here I am!

This interview illustrates how little is said by the interviewing
dentist in contrast to the large amount of information provided
freely by the patient. The patient has described her confusion, her
attitudes concerning dentistry, her desire to have a healthy mouth,
and an apparent lack of support from her husband concerning her
dental problems. She is discouraged and somewhat angry, anxious,
and depressed. She has tried her best to take care of her mouth,
dreads the thought of losing her teeth, and yet finds herself facing
more dental treatments and efforts to follow preventive dental
care recommendations. The expression of these feelings to an attentive, understanding listener was the first step in forming a
therapeutic relationship.

This interview concluded with a review of the previously completed questionnaire and a few brief comments by the interviewing
dentist concerning the relationship of diabetes and periodontal
disease. The information provided by the patient during the interview enabled the dentist to make recommendations for treatment
and preventive care that were compatible with the patient's emotional needs and attitudes.

Patient 2. Mr. P. is a forty-year-old self-employed truck operator.
He is very concerned about loss of income when he doesn't work.
Appointments for dental treatment interfere with his work schedule. During the interview, the patient spoke rapidly and spent
most of the time sitting on the edge of his chair.

DOCTOR: Tell me, what brings you in this morning?
PATIENT: Right here in the front lower teeth I've got white pus.
I've had it for a good many years. Every time I go to a dentist I
always ask, "Are you ever going to take care of that?" but it never
gets taken care of. I'm in the trucking business and my time is
very valuable. This visit is costing me a lot of money, but I finally
came to a point where I've just got to have somebody look at it.
I don't think it's anything major, but I could be wrong. I brush,
I floss, but I still have white pus. That's why I came in: to see

what could be done about it. And I really need to have my teeth cleaned. So these two things have brought me to your office. My wife wanted me to come in, too. It looks to me as if the gum is getting progressively worse as the years go on, I guess. I'm here to find out if I'm doing something wrong or if this can be prevented or controlled by treatment.

DOCTOR: You say your gums are looking worse?

PATIENT: Well, it seems that in the last two years if I don't brush my teeth really well, the pus will just pop up. That didn't happen before. That's the thing that concerns me. It doesn't seem that I have problems any other place.

DOCTOR: How do you feel about going to the dentist?

PATIENT: I have no qualms about that. The only thing that irritates me is that it's very hard for me to take those mouth x-rays. I choke and gag! You know how they always jam that film in your mouth and say "Don't move" and "Don't breathe"; I have a very difficult time doing that. Once when I had my whole mouth full of plaster of paris, whew, boy! I didn't think I'd make it through that. When I do go to a dentist I don't worry about money. If I need something fixed, fix it. Don't fix one tooth today, one tomorrow, and one the day after. If I've got four cavities, I want them all fixed, one pop, and be done with it. I like to get things rolling. Money is not the problem; time is. I want them all fixed today, one pop!

The interview continued in the same manner. The patient repeated his desire for "all treatment in one pop!" and became more impatient as the conversation proceeded. Although under pressure from the patient, the dentist did not hurry the interview, rush the clinical examination, or compromise the recommended treatment. By learning of the patient's extreme concern for time, the dentist was able to convince him that preventive measures such as daily use of dental floss, though time-consuming, would markedly reduce future needs for lengthy dental treatment appointments, thus enhancing his strongest motivation. The dentist also made efforts to perform the needed treatment in as few appointments as possible.

Patients Who Provoke Anxiety in the Dentist

It is necessary for the dentist to remain under emotional control during the interview. Patients who make provocative statements, express anger and hostility, cry, or question the doctor's knowledge and skills make the interviewing dentist feel uncomfortable.

When feeling anxious or threatened, the dentist may attempt to establish control of the situation and of the patient in a variety of ways, such as exerting authority, changing the subject, or terminating the interview. These actions are inappropriate because they halt the flow of potentially useful information. By remaining under personal control and responding appropriately to the patient's anxiety-provoking behavior, the interview can usually continue. An excerpt from an interview with a hostile patient is presented here.

Patient 3. Mrs. K., the forty-two-year-old wife of a physician, spent much of the first part of the interview asking the dentist questions about his academic background and practice experience. She related a number of anecdotes reflecting authority conflicts with physicians, dentists, and veterinarians and emphasized her feelings that their role was to make recommendations and her prerogative was to decide which recommendations to follow. The interviewing dentist became more anxious and tense as the interview proceeded. He made an effort to gain control of the situation by impressing the patient with his status and his understanding of her psychological makeup.

> DOCTOR: With what you've been saying, it sounds as if you don't relate well to doctors who use their authority; doctors who tell you what to do and won't let you be involved in what's going on.
> PATIENT: Of course! How many times do I have to say it? I'm entitled to my opinions. Just because you're a doctor, that doesn't mean you can tell me what to do.
> DOCTOR: Okay. Now, have any of your previous dentists discussed with you the causes of gum troubles or tooth decay and why people get these conditions?

PATIENT: Well . . . I'm not sure anybody really knows. From all the reading I've done, it looks like the dentists aren't really sure.

DOCTOR: No, there's been some very significant research that has shown . . .

Here followed a brief "lecture" on the nature of dental disease. The interview ended at this point, with the patient and the dentist at a standoff; neither would yield to the other's authority. Needless to say, an effective relationship was not established.

Patient 4. Mrs. J., thirty-three years old, reported regular visits for dental treatment but expressed a vague suspicion that much of her past dental care had been inadequate. She fidgeted nervously throughout the interview. The interviewing dentist found that his efforts to facilitate communication were not successful. The patient's comments were anecdotal, seemingly unrelated, and often highly critical of the dental profession. In an effort to bring the interview into a pertinent context, the dentist resorted prematurely to direct questioning. As is shown by the following brief excerpt, the anxious dentist's leading and suggestive questions led the interview down a blind alley.

DOCTOR: Have you had any bad experiences with dentists or dentistry in the past?

PATIENT: No.

DOCTOR: Have you had any problems? A lot of people come here and the first thing they say is, "I'm really afraid, I don't want to be here."

PATIENT: Yes. I don't want to be here.

DOCTOR: Have you had fears or anxieties before in going to the dentist for regular care?

PATIENT: Yes. I don't like to go. I don't like pain. I'd much rather go to a medical doctor than to a dentist. Don't ask me why!

At this point the dentist was not able to get the interview process restarted. He began a rapid review of the questionnaire before performing the clinical examination. An open-ended inquiry concerning past dental experiences, such as, "Tell me about your past dental care," would have been appropriate, facilitative, and probably effective in gaining the needed information.

Dental Emergency Patients

The dental emergency patient poses a special problem for the interviewer. Such a patient is usually in pain and under stress. Frequently, the emergency patient has not been cared for by the dentist he comes to with the emergency. Furthermore, the professional staff may view his treatment as a disruption in the office schedule. In addition, many such patients ask for symptomatic relief only and have no apparent interest in remedial or preventive care. Nevertheless, the dentist needs some information about the patient's problem, his previous dental care, and his general health in order to provide treatment for the emergency.

The dentist usually "squeezes" emergency patients into his schedule. As a result, he has little time available for their treatment. This, plus the patient's pain and stress, frequently make it impossible to carry out a detailed, open-ended interview. It is still essential to give the patient an opportunity to express feelings about his problems. An abbreviated interview, in an open-ended style, will elicit the essential data and help to reduce the patient's anxiety. If the attitudes of the dentist and the clinical staff indicate compassion and interest in the patient, he may accept recommendations for complete dental evaluation and treatment after the urgent problem has been resolved.

Patient. 5. This is an example of an interview with an emergency patient. It was carried out in a teratment room.

DOCTOR: Good morning, Mrs. ———. I'm Dr. ———. How may I help you today?

PATIENT: My tooth, right here, has been hurting for three days!

DOCTOR: Three days?

PATIENT: Yes, and it's getting worse.

DOCTOR: Have you ever had a problem like this before?

PATIENT: Only once about two years ago.

DOCTOR: What was done for you then?

PATIENT: The dentist pulled my tooth.

DOCTOR: I'm sorry to hear that you lost a tooth. What do you think might have to be done for the toothache you now have?

PATIENT: I hope the tooth doesn't need pulling. I fainted the last time.

DOCTOR: Fainted the last time?

The patient went on to tell about fainting for a short time when given an injection of local anesthetic. The questionnaire did not reveal significant past or present medical illnesses. The dentist asked a few direct questions about the nature of the tooth pain in order to begin developing a differential diagnosis and then proceeded to examine her mouth. The total elapsed time for this short interview was approximately five minutes.

Review of Health History Questionnaires

During the latter part of a patient interview, the interviewer should begin to exert more control and ask direct questions of the patient. The interviewer may conclude the interview by reviewing a health history questionnaire previously completed by the patient. Thus, toward the end of the interview the interviewer can deal with very specific information.

Patient 6. The following example illustrates the use of direct questioning and facilitation during questionnaire review with a patient. Note how the use of open-ended interviewing techniques produced information that goes well beyond the patient's written responses on the questionnaire. The patient was a thirty-five-year-old man.

DOCTOR: Okay, may I ask a couple of specific questions related to the questionnaire that we had you fill out? You gave a "yes" answer to having your teeth ground to improve your bite. What was that about?

PATIENT: I wasn't really too sure about that. I know that the dentist

took a mouth impression when he was putting in that bridge. I
don't remember if he actually ground my teeth, but he was fitting
these teeth in the bridge into my bite. Maybe I made an incorrect statement on the questionnaire.

DOCTOR: Now I understand what went on. I see you've written a
note here: "wisdom teeth."

PATIENT: I have had some weird experiences with wisdom teeth!

DOCTOR: Weird experiences?

PATIENT: Every one of them swelled up like an apple and just (*snaps
fingers*) like that. One time, years ago, I was at a race and within
twenty minutes my mouth was as big as an apple. Every one of
them, all four, did exactly the same thing.

DOCTOR: You mean before they were taken out they got infected?

PATIENT: Yes, they just blew up. I'd feel a little twinge, and within
a half an hour my jaw would be like an apple.

DOCTOR: How did you do after they were removed?

PATIENT: No problem!

Sometimes even the most skilled dental interviewer will not obtain
relevant health information during the interview. Many patients
do not associate past or current medical problems with dental
treatment and fail to discuss them with the dentist. A questionnaire may uncover health problems that are possibly related to
dental care. The following example demonstrates direct facilitation, questioning, and confrontation during a questionnaire review
with a patient.

Patient 7. The patient, a twenty-eight-year-old woman, appeared
relaxed and friendly throughout the interview.

DOCTOR: I note that you didn't answer "yes" or "no" to the question about fainting spells or convulsions.

PATIENT: No.

DOCTOR: The answer is "no"?

PATIENT: No, I just didn't answer the question.

DOCTOR: Have you ever had fainting spells or convulsions?

PATIENT: Uh . . . I'm not sure . . . I mean . . .

DOCTOR: You seem upset that I'm asking you this.

PATIENT: Well, I just don't understand what that has to do with getting my teeth fixed!

The dentist responded by describing the possibility that drugs used in treating convulsive disorders might affect the health of the gums. In addition, he expressed the concern that a convulsive seizure during dental treatment might be hazardous to a patient. The interview then continued.

PATIENT: I'm sorry I didn't understand. It's just that I've always been sort of embarrassed about it.
DOCTOR: I understand.
PATIENT: I've had a few fainting spells since I was nine. I take medication every day to prevent them.

This information gave the dentist an important understanding of the patient's medical problem and feelings and enabled him to provide effective treatment safeguards and appropriate support for her.

4 SPECIAL INTERVIEWING SITUATIONS IN DENTAL PRACTICE

Interviewing Families, Children, and Adolescents

It is often advantageous in dental practice to have more than one family member participate in an interview. Successful dental treatment may depend upon changes in a patient's life style or habits, such as eliminating sugar from the diet or giving up smoking. The dentist may ask the patient to perform difficult tooth-cleaning procedures at home. The patient may have to make important financial decisions concerning proposed dental treatment. If the dentist incorrectly views the patient as an isolated individual, certain professional recommendations may be doomed to failure owing to lack of support from the patient's family.

By interviewing children or adolescents and parents together, much information can be gained about family interactions. This knowledge can be essential in planning treatment for the young patient, predicting compliance with preventive or nutritional recommendations, and assessing the patient's relationship to authority figures. Resistance to parental authority may be manifested as failure to comply with dental treatment recommendations. By interviewing teenagers and parents together, dysfunctional relationships among them may become evident. This will, in turn, enable the therapist to plan a strategy of treatment that emphasizes mutual cooperation. After the family interview has been concluded, adolescents and older children can be separated from the parents and the interview continued with the young patient. This emphasizes the younger patient's individuality and enables the clinician to gain information in a situation less influenced by the presence of a parent.

By interviewing husbands and wives toegther, one can often prevent problems in dental practice. Patient 1, discussed earlier in this section, expressed dismay that she was "the one that's ending up with all the gum disease and [her husband] really doesn't care." If she arrived home to discuss with her husband an extensive treatment plan and a substantial professional fee, she might have found him unwilling to provide financial support for her treatment. However, if the dentist invites the spouse to participate in the initial interview and hear recommendations in a discussion of findings, the dentist can help prevent many problems that result from inadequate family communication. Additional information about techniques of interviewing children, families, and informants is presented in Chapters 6 and 8.

Interviewing and Continuing Dental Care

The initial open-ended interview establishes a pattern of communication that should continue between dentists, patients, and staff members throughout future dental care. Dental staff can utilize basic interviewing techniques, modified to reflect a continuing relationship, during the patient's treatment appointments and periodic evaluations. The role of the interview in continuing care is discussed in more detail in Chapter 11.

Continuing communication nurtures the mutual trust developed during an initial series of interviews. Such trust will assist the practitioner of dentistry when he finds it necessary to refer a patient to a specialist. Patients accept threatening referrals, such as referrals to psychiatrists, oral surgeons, or periodontists, more readily when they are given an opportunity to participate in the decision to seek further help and to discuss their feelings in the matter.

The dentist who uses the techniques of the open-ended interview in practice will find that many of the stresses associated with dental practice are diminished. If staff members are provided with the opportunity to become familiar with interviewing principles, they, too, will be able to deal more effectively with the stresses and anxieties experienced by them and by patients. When all people who meet patients are able to communicate effectively and listen to them with sensitivity and understanding, "going to the dentist" becomes more rewarding for patients and clinicians alike.

10

DISCUSSING FINDINGS AND PLANNING TREATMENT

1   DISCUSSING THE FINDINGS

At the conclusion of a diagnostic interview, the patient expects to be given a summary of the findings. In most instances, he will want to know about the prognosis, whether treatment is to follow, and what it will be. There are exceptions, of course. Some patients do not want the responsibility of sharing knowledge of the nature of the problem, nor do they wish to have any responsibility in the treatment. They may even try to prevent a discussion of the findings and planning of treatment. Others will want to know as much as possible, often more than the physician knows at that point. In all cases, however, the interview should be terminated in such a way that further studies, if needed, or treatment procedures, if they are to begin now, can be carried out successfully. This means involving the patient responsibly in a collaboration.

The Discussion

The discussion should open with a frank and clear statement of what the physician has found, in sufficient detail to give the patient an understanding of the problem. The significance of the findings should be explained. At this time, too, the physician should describe the areas of uncertainty for which more data is needed and describe what must be done next, such as laboratory tests, other diagnostic procedures, and further observation.

A common error in this phase of the interview is the use of medical parlance in presenting the information. Ordinary, non-technical language should be used and simple analogies employed to clarify physiological processes being discussed. Vocabulary appropriate to the person's socio-economic status and education should be used. A particular problem faces the clinician in explaining findings to a patient who is from a culture with which he is unfamiliar, who uses an idiom that is foreign to the physician (such as the ghetto black or the chicano), or who has a rudimentary grasp of English.

A complete discussion of the findings does not, however, mean overloading the patient with information. Findings of dubious relevance should be omitted. Throughout the explanation, the physician must be alert to the patient's response to ensure that his explanation is being understood.

There are many patients who consider it impolite to interrupt the physician, to ask questions, or to reveal that they did not understand the explanation that was given. In a study of doctor-patient communication done at Michigan State University, a well-mannered, smiling, middle-class widow in her sixties was given a deliberately over-detailed and confusing explanation by her physician. Throughout the explanation, she nodded in polite agreement, occasionally echoing a word or phrase, and said, "Thank you, doctor," at the conclusion. The physician then asked, "Now, do you understand Mrs. R.?" "Oh, yes, doctor," she replied sweetly and respectfully. Gently, but insistently, he said, "What did I just tell you?" She blushed and became quite embarrassed. Only with difficulty was she able to admit that she had become lost very early in the explanation.

The lesson in this is that one cannot be sure from the patient's manner alone that he has understood your explanation or your instructions. At the conclusion, it is necessary to inquire.

An inquiry about the patient's feelings and any questions he may have is also necessary, since, first of all, any explanation, discussion, or recommendation relating to illness will evoke some anxiety and perhaps a mixture of emotions in response. Second, unless they are very passive or handle anxiety by denial, patients will almost always have some further questions. The inquiry should begin in an open-ended way, perhaps something like an encouraging gesture inviting the patient to speak. If facilitation fails to elicit a response, the physician can ask directly, "How do you feel about this?" It is important to permit the patient to express his anxiety, worry, or any other emotional response he might have and to encourage him if he has difficulty expressing it.

When a patient does express his feelings, the most appropriate response from the physician is support. This gives the patient the comfort of knowing he has a concerned physician. Of course, if the patient expresses fear that is unrealistic, that is, about which the physician can honestly give reassurance, he should do so.

Some patients who express their feelings of fear and concern when encouraged to do so may hesitate to ask questions. Blum points out that clinic patients, in particular, rarely ask for detailed information about their condition, and that the less general information a patient has, the less he will ask for. He comments,

> The self-perpetuation of ignorance on the part of the patient who does not ask the doctor any questions is probably related to cultural, social class, and personality factors. It is reasonable to expect that the more the patient views the doctor as a stranger in language, custom, or outlook, then the less likely will the patient be to begin conversation. It is also likely that the more the patient is afraid of the doctor, or the more inferior the patient feels to the doctor, the less likely will the patient be to ask questions. The regrettable consequence is that communication problems will be greatest with people who need the information the most: people from different cultures, the lower class, or unreasonable and uncooperative people.[1]

Having, therefore, described his findings in clear and non-technical terms; indicated areas of uncertainty and of insufficient information, and what further procedures may be needed; clarified, as much as the information at hand permits, the significance of the findings; facilitated expression of the patient's feelings and responded supportively; the physician must find out if the patient understands. Does he remember what the physician has said? Is it clear to him? The physician should never fail, at this point, to ask, "Do you have any questions?" If the patient does not understand what his situation really is, he will be unable to participate responsibly in his treatment.

The Patient's Response

Patients' responses to the discussion of findings vary considerably. Some responses represent an attempt to shut off communication. The healthiest response is, of course, a desire to know the situation. Blum[2] describes a few characteristic responses that make for management problems if not dealt with effectively. He calls these: "I don't want to know, so don't tell me," "reassure me," and "prove your love." To these we would add the counterphobic response and overdone "good and reasonable" behavior.

I Don't Want to Know, So Don't Tell Me

This statement may be made directly by the patient or expressed in his attitude, in which case the patient is not hearing what the doctor says though he may superficially appear attentive. It comes from patients who are fearful of taking responsibility for their future, preferring instead to depend entirely on the physician. This response makes it difficult to carry out treatment successfully. Accompanied by a certain amount of flattery of the doctor, if not overdone it may lull him into overlooking the attitude and failing to deal with it by confronting the patient. The physician now may be maneuvered into the position of protecting his patient from reality and encouraging the patient's dependency. In such cases, after confronting the patient with his behavior, it is often possible to engage him more responsibly in his treatment.

Reassure Me

The plea for reassurance, as Blum points out, is an invitation to make a promise which, though reducing the patient's fear of an unfavorable outcome, may be impossible to keep. While an honest reassurance in the form of a conservatively phrased prediction can allay anxiety, this sort of prediction often cannot be made after the initial diagnostic examination. This may be because more data are needed, or it may be that the outcome is in doubt and could be unfavorable. In any event, support is more important than reassurance at this point, even when reassurance is honestly given. The clinician should clearly express his ability to appreciate how the patient must feel, his concern, and his intent that all possible appropriate diagnostic and treatment procedures be brought to bear on the problem. Reassurance tends to cut off further communication from the patient about his fears or worries, with a risk of giving the doctor an unwarranted feeling that he has solved the problem of the patient's apprehensiveness.

Prove Your Love

Jokes are made about the physician's instructions to the patient to go to bed, take two aspirins every four hours, and drink plenty of fluids. They reflect the fact that many patients are disappointed if they don't get some medicine or a "shot." The "prove your love" response, often expressed in a disappointed, "Aren't you going to give me some medicine?"—a request for visible proof of the doctor's concern for the patient—is most likely to occur when simple, supportive measures or no medication is indicated.

There are physicians who regularly give antibiotics for upper respiratory infections, whether or not they are indicated, to "prove their love" and to satisfy the patient. Others use vitamins or minor tranquilizers this way. Still others deliberately prescribe placebos. In our opinion placebos should be used with great discrimination. It is true that some patients reason primitively and cannot grasp that they can be appropriately cared for even though no medication is given. But most patients respond positively to a sensible discussion that shows respect for their intelligence, and there is then no need for pretense in the form of placebos. We don't want to "addict" patients to medical care and to unnecessary medications, nor to suggest that an answer to all discomfort can be found in a pill or a "shot." Many a drug-dependent individual has been trained to be so by a physician who used his prescription pad too freely. The capacity for self-help and knowledge about when it is appropriate to consult the health care professional cannot be cultivated by prescribing placebos. Educating patients about medication and its overuse is an important part of patient care.

Counterphobic Response

This is a variation on the theme of "I don't want to know, so don't tell me." The patient's fears are similar, but his response is to deny that he is ill or needs help." "Nonsense," he says, "I'm not ill, nor am I helpless. I don't need you at all." His anxiety that illness could result in helplessness is so sharp that he will behave in ways that demonstrate to himself and others that he is far from helpless. These are the patients who ignore the doctor's advice and prefer do-it-yourself medical care. Breaking through this defensive wall is possible when the patient has consulted you on his own initiative. Confronting him with his attitude makes a realistic discussion possible. If he is reluctantly following another's advice, or has involuntarily become your patient because of a medical emergency, it is very difficult to get him to recognize his underlying anxiety. Whenever possible, the clinician should aim to make the patient aware of his attitude through confrontation given supportively, and he should help the patient express his anxiety. This can lead to a realistic discussion of the patient's situation.

Overdone "Good and Reasonable" Behavior

Some patients who are frightened of illness take a "good child" stance when threatened by it. They make no demands, express no fear, and behave as though the physician were unusually skilled and unquestionably able to banish illness. They respond, verbally and non-verbally, with, "Anything you say, doctor. I fear nothing because you are my doctor. I will make no demands on you and will follow your orders completely." Such patients are afraid that to burden the physician with their apprehensions and concerns will annoy him. They feel that they can influence him to exert all his magic and rescue them if he really likes them. As a result, their psychological distress is not relieved because they are afraid to communicate their fears. Fear is usually reduced by the simple measure of expressing it to another in a helping relationship. When the physician thinks of such a patient as a "good" patient because of this obedient attitude, he may fail to help the patient express and face his anxiety.

This is why the physician must be alert to the patient's verbal and non-verbal response and identify it even as it is happening. This is another way of saying that the task of data collection and evaluation is not discontinued during the discussion of findings and planning of treatment. Rather, observation of the verbal and non-verbal cues about the nature of the patient's response should be a primary concern during the discussion. If the patient is distressed and responds in one or more of the ways described above, the physician should discuss his feelings with him. The physician's task is to help the patient accept the reality of his situation, to help him make a realistic appraisal of it, to permit him the opportunity to voice his concerns, and to help him begin to deal constructively with the situation.

2   PLANNING TREATMENT

When more data must be gathered—by laboratory or radiological studies, for instance—the patient should be presented with a clear plan for future action. This will be discussed in detail later in this chapter.

When there is sufficient data and treatment can proceed, the physician's instructions should be equally clear and detailed. And it is quite important that the patient's involvement is such that "getting well" is the mutual aim of physician and patient. The patient, in other words, should share the physician's therapeutic goals, understand their respective roles in the treatment, and be prepared to be a responsible partner in the undertaking.

An approach some physicians use in attempting to motivate their patients is to frighten them into following their instructions carefully. This is always an error. Fear makes people less capable of listening and remembering. This was well demonstrated by a study of fear-arousing communication,[3] in which a fifteen-minute illustrated lecture was prepared in three forms, all containing the same essential information about causes of tooth decay and the same recommendations about oral hygiene. One contained a very strong cautionary appeal emphasizing such unpleasant consequences of bad dental habits as pain, advanced gum disease, secondary illnesses, and ugly teeth; and it was made personal (that is, "*This* could happen to you"). The moderate appeal presented the same information less stridently, and the minimal appeal rarely alluded to the consequences of tooth neglect. The subjects were divided into three groups, each of which heard one of the lectures. Their immediate and later responses were studied. The strong appeal aroused the greatest emotional response; however, the attitudes and oral hygiene practices of the group who heard the minimal appeal had changed within one week, while neither changed in the strong appeal group. One year later a follow-up questionnaire indicated that conformity to the recommended practices was still significantly higher in the minimal than in the strong appeal group. There was evidence that the strong appeal had aroused fear and anger, followed by a defensive avoidance of the internal and external cues that were present when the fear was aroused. In other words, frightening the subjects in the experiment had "turned them off."

It is better to take an educational approach. This means a clear and informative discussion, in non-technical language, of the treatment aims and the relationship of each part of the treatment plan to the treatment goals. Once it is clear that the patient understands and accepts the aims, the clinician can proceed with directions. But getting commitment from the patient to those aims is the most important single factor in assuring that he will follow directions.

To clarify whether the patient understands the treatment plan and is committed to it and to the goals of treatment, it is well for the physician to ask him to summarize what he will do. In order for the patient to restate the physician's recommendations, he must understand them. The physician can reinforce them by writing them out for the patient.

3   SPECIAL PROBLEMS

I Don't Know

Probably the most difficult situation for both physician and patient is when the diagnosis, and consequently future treatment, is unclear. This may be the case because the total amount of information about the problem is inadequate, or because the physician's skill and knowledge are inadequate to make maximal use of the available information. In the first instance, more information may be sought. It may be, however, that the patient's problem has not evolved far enough in its biological course to reveal diagnostic clues; necessary information may not yet be available. In the second instance, a consultant with specialized skills and knowledge may be brought in.

It is important to clarify which of the two situations obtains in any instance, as they call for very different approaches. Though the liberal use of consultation has much to recommend it, except in those cases where consultation is urgently needed, problems may be created if it is called for too early—that is, before a firm doctor-patient relationship has been established. This may lead to a premature and inaccurate judgment about the physician's skills, and a good relationship of mutual trust and cooperation may never be reached. Lines of communication and areas of responsibility between primary physician, consultant, and patient may become confused. The patient's anxiety may be raised by the inference that consultation means a serious or life-threatening disease. And one must be reasonably certain that consultation will help, as it may be both expensive and futile if, in fact, the problem is undiagnosable.

As stated before, a clear plan for future action is called for when a diagnosis cannot yet be reached. This should include a direct admission, without evasiveness, that a diagnosis has not yet been made, a statement of what has been learned, and a description of the plan for observation and further study. If possible, an estimate should be given of the length of time required to make a definite diagnosis. If symptomatic therapy is to be carried on in the interval, its purpose (to control discomfort) should be stated. The primary objective of this discussion with the patient is to establish that he is not being abandoned, that the physician remains concerned, will see him regularly and be alertly observant, and that the physician is prepared to act promptly when the situation changes.

If uncertainty persists for more than a few weeks, the patient will require increasing reassurance and support. Though the physician should indicate concern, it is important to avoid communicating anxiety to the patient. An unpublished study of a group of patients by Greene and Swisher indicated that major problems of patient management, including breakdown of the doctor-patient relationship and serious psychological distress in the patient or physician, occur more commonly in the situation of indeterminacy and indecision than in the management of the severely or fatally ill patient.

Referrals

If the physician decides that consultation is needed, he should discuss it with the patient. Preparation for a consultation is an important part of patient care; unfortunately it is omitted in far too many cases. Considerable anxiety in patients could be avoided if this matter were given more attention.

The referring physician should describe his reasons for requesting consultation, what procedures the patient will undergo, and what will follow. If it is clear that a number of visits to the consultant will be required, the physician should say so. Similarly, the referring physician should give the consultant a complete report of his findings and state his reasons for requesting consultation and what he expects from it.

Some delicacy is required in referring a patient to a psychiatrist for consultation or possible treatment. The patient may have a variety of fears and concerns and often a good deal of resistance

to the idea. A single discussion with the patient may not be sufficient. After a tactful description of the reasons for the referral, it
is important that the physician encourage the patient to express
his concerns or questions and to deal with them factually but supportively. Frequent questions that arise are: "Do you mean I'm
imagining this?" "Does this mean I'm not really sick?" "Do you
think I'm mentally ill?" Making a successful referral in this case
depends on taking enough time to deal with such questions and
concerns.

"Do you think I'm imagining this?" calls for a firm and clear
"No." This should be followed by a simple and non-technical explanation of the clinician's concept of the relationship between
the evidence of psychological difficulties (such as anxiety, depression, or family conflicts, for example) and the symptoms experienced by the patient. Simple psycho-physiological mechanisms can
be described where appropriate, such as the relationship between
anxiety and heart rate, or depression and general psychomotor re-
tardation. Questions about mental illness require that the clinician
find out what the patient's concept of mental illness is. When
these are related to a memory of a senile relative or a psychotic
family member, one is usually in a position to be honestly reassuring. Again, a description of the relationship between emotional
conflict and its consequences, on the one hand, and physiological
symptoms, on the other, can be helpful. When the reason for referral is that evidence from the interview and mental status examination indicate that the patient might be psychotic, tact is essential. "I think you do have mental and emotional problems, but I
think Dr. B_____ may be able to help you" emphasizes the positive element of the potential for help in the consultation rather
than the labeling. In some cases, more than one appointment with
the patient may be necessary before the patient will accept a psychiatric referral.

Fatal Illness

When the findings indicate a high probability of fatal illness, the
physician is likely to feel some conflict about how to discuss this.

How much should he tell? Should the facts be presented to the patient, to the family, or to both?

The response of the patient and the patient's family is likely to vary with the diagnosis. The diagnosis of cancer or leukemia, for example, is usually received with an expectation of a downhill course and a slow, painful death. On the other hand, a myocardial infarction in a patient with severe coronary arteriosclerosis has the same prognosis, but patients rarely feel the same despair about it. Chronic progressive respiratory insufficiency associated with severe pulmonary fibrosis has an inexorably downhill course, but, again, does not usually evoke the pessimism and despondency that attends the diagnosis of cancer.

The initial response of some patients who are told they have cancer is denial ("This can't be happening to me"), followed by a reactive depression. Some become openly angry. Young adults with family responsibilities are most likely to be angry and bitter at first and then be more open about their depression. Care of the patient with fatal illness is discussed in detail in Chapter 11.

The discussion of the findings and planning of treatment sets the tone for the clinician-patient relationship that will guide the patient's care for the duration of the illness. Hopefully it will establish an atmosphere that promotes good care in health and illness for some time to come. The next chapter describes interviewing in the continuing care of patients.

REFERENCES

1. Blum, R. H., *The Management of the Doctor-Patient Relationship.* New York: McGraw-Hill, 1960, p. 127.
2. Ibid., pp. 179-183.
3. Hovland, C. L., I. L. Janis, and H. H. Kelley, *Communication and Persuasion.* New Haven: Yale University Press, 1953.

11

INTERVIEWING AND CONTINUING CARE

Interviewing is perhaps the most important element in the continuing care of patients. Once established, the ideal clinician-patient relationship as defined in Chapter 2 requires continuing attention to interviewing. If the clinician can maintain good communication with the patient, he will be perceived as an ally and a resource for guidance in those aspects of the patient's life that affect his health and well-being. Effective interviewing also facilitates compliance with treatment and the planning of rehabilitation.

After an initial diagnostic interview or series of interviews, the clinician and patient discuss the findings and plan of treatment (see Chapter 10). Careful interviewing, however, does not stop there. Maintaining open communication is necessary to monitor progress and to achieve effective therapy. The clinician-patient relationship must be nurtured. It is affected by changes in the patient's health status, including improvement or deterioration of the patient's condition during the course of the illness. Drug side-effects or a new illness may also affect the relationship. The patient's willingness to take prescribed medications and to follow other treatment recommendations (e.g., diets, exercise) partly depends on his rapport with the clinician. Indeed, even the patient's perception of his progress is influenced by how he feels about the clinician. In this chapter we will discuss interviewing in terms of the ongoing office patient, the care of the healthy patient, the care and follow-up of patients in which the diagnosis is unknown or uncertain, the continuing care of patients with chronic disease, and the care of the dying patient.

THE ONGOING OFFICE PATIENT

Many patients see the physician regularly because of a chronic, relatively stable illness such as hypertension or cerebrovascular disease. Ideally, the interview should be allotted at least half of the time scheduled to be spent with the patient. It is important to inquire about the impact of the illness on the patient's life. What is its effect on the quality of the patient's life? What are his feelings about the necessary restrictions imposed on him by the treatment regimen? Compliance with the treatment recommendations is greatly facilitated when these matters are openly discussed. The clinician may be aware of the patient's difficulties but not of his perception of them. The medical concerns of the physician may not coincide with the concerns of the patient, or they may not have the same priority to the patient.

A common problem in medical practice is the patient with essential hypertension.

L.S. is a seventy-one-year-old Caucasian widow. She has led her employer to believe she is ten years younger than her actual age so she can continue to work. She has stable angina, but during a routine office visit she mentions that substernal pain is awakening her at night. She was obviously apprehensive and wanted gastrointestinal studies. She was reluctant to have a treadmill test of cardiac function when the physician suggested that it would be most appropriate.

L.S.: Doctor, are all these tests really necessary? I really don't have time.

DOCTOR: What time commitments do you have?

L.S.: I have to be at work by 10 A.M. Then, I have to catch the bus at 4:15 P.M. to be home by 4:45 so I can help my sister with dinner. God forbid she should have to start dinner alone.

DOCTOR: You live with your sister?

L.S.: For the last five years. I'm all she's got, and because she doesn't do anything else, I'm her whole day. She can drive me crazy by the end of a weekend. Thank God for my job; it gets me out of the house.

DOCTOR: Your job sounds very important to you.

L.S.: I really don't like to miss time from my job—if I lost it, I don't know what I'd do. I never want to retire—I like being active. It's my contact with normal people. If I had to spend every day with my sister, I know I couldn't take it.

DOCTOR: I can see how important your work is to you. Think about this: if I treat your stomach without being certain of what's wrong, your illness could be prolonged. If we do the tests now, I know exactly what to treat and in the long run you'll miss less work.

L.S. (*after a reflective moment of silence*): Okay, doc. But don't find anything really wrong, please!

DOCTOR: From what you tell me, I think it's still early enough to treat whatever we might find.

By facilitating the expression of the patient's apprehensions and concerns, the physician was able to avoid an unnecessary procedure and proceed with appropriate studies.

When a patient who has been previously diagnosed and treated returns to the office with a new complaint, the clinician must look beyond the immediate problem of concern to the patient. The apparent problem is often only the patient's ticket of admission to the doctor's office. One should be aware that the initial complaint may mask other, more serious problems. Typical complaints are headaches, fatigue, lack of pep, accidental injuries, or minor infections. The clinician should ask himself, "Why is the illness happening now?" Other questions to be considered are: "What were the circumstances surrounding the accident?" "What was going on in the patient's life when the infection occurred?" A large number of orthopedic and burn injuries are associated with alcohol or drug abuse. Many headaches are caused by musculoskeletal contractions due to tension. The most common cause of fatigue or lack of pep is depression.

A thirty-one-year-old single woman came to the doctor's office complaining of a sore throat and swollen glands. She appeared to have a bacterial or viral infection and wanted treatment with an antibiotic. She asked if the medication the physician might prescribe could interfere with birth control. In answer to a question on this point, she responded that she was considering taking birth control pills since her boyfriend had just moved in with her. Further, because she considered herself physically unattractive, she had recently lost weight through dieting for the first time in her life. She wished to enter a sexual relationship with her boyfriend but lacked self-confidence, especially about her ability to perform sexually. Obviously, the correct therapy involved much more than the antibiotic she originally sought.

DOCTOR: Are you now taking birth control pills?

K.S.: No. My boyfriend has just moved in and I've been thinking about getting them.

DOCTOR: Are you and your boyfriend sexually active?

K.S.: No, not yet. I'm too embarrassed. At night I sleep in one bed on one side of the room and he sleeps in the other.

DOCTOR: You're embarrassed?

K.S.: Yeah. At night I cover myself up completely in the bed—even my head—and pretend to be asleep when he comes out of the bathroom, so I don't have to talk or deal with the issue. I don't want him to see my body. I used to be fat, and about a year and a half ago I lost a lot of weight. I had a boyfriend for about two weeks last year, but this is my first real relationship. I know I stayed fat so I would always be unattractive and not have to deal with this. My girlfriends are real encouraging, and I'm better than I used to be, but I'm scared.

DOCTOR: But now you'd like to pursue things with this man?

K.S.: Very much. I know it's just a matter of time till we sleep together. He wants to already, and I guess I should be prepared.

The patient was able to express her real concerns when the clinician looked beyond her manifest concerns.

THE CARE OF THE HEALTHY PATIENT

In many instances the patient who comes to see a clinician has no illness, as when a person comes for an annual physical examination. In such cases, the interviewer should inquire about the pattern of health and illness over the previous year. This can be done with an open-ended inquiry such as, "What has been happening since your last visit?" The interview should also include a more structured inquiry into the patient's history since the last visit, including medications, drug side-effects, and visits to other physicians or health care specialists. The patient may have a new chief complaint or a list of small problems saved up over the past year. The clinician should try to assess the relative importance the patient attaches to each of them.

A useful question in assessing the well patient's health and quality of life is to ask him to describe a typical day in his life. Routines and behavior patterns to which the patient no longer gives conscious thought may have an impact on his health. They may also reflect the emergence of a new health problem. After a general, open-ended inquiry, the clinician should inquire into such specifics as sleeping, eating, and work schedule if these things have not been spontaneously described. Another appropriate area for inquiry is work, including what the patient enjoys and what is stressful. The clinician should watch carefully for expressions of emotion or lack of it as the patient describes his day. Attention should be given to body language and facial expressions during the account. One may ask about leisure activities, including time spent with family, time spent alone, exercise, and the patient's attitude toward all of these. Opening up these areas promotes the discussion of health behavior. It is important to discuss the adverse effects of smoking, drinking, and recreational drug abuse when the patient has described such behavior. When a patient is ill, his motivation to change his health-related behavior is high. When there is no immediate threat to health, the motivation to change is low. Developing a "wellness program" in the interview with a healthy patient can increase motivation to change behavior that is potentially dangerous to health.

W.V. is a fifty-two-year-old lawyer. His father died of a heart attack at the age of fifty-five. The patient smokes one pack of cigarettes a day, which he believes helps him to handle stress. He would like to stop but fears gaining weight. In a discussion of his risk of heart disease, he expresses concern but has no long-term health enhancement goals. Directed inquiry reveals that he enjoys swimming and finds it relaxing, though he swims infrequently. His wife is willing to join him in a program of fitness built around daily swimming.

Some patients request a complete physical examination to "rule out disease." The patient will often say, "I just want to be certain there isn't anything really wrong with me." This should be a signal to the clinician that the patient has something else on his mind. The patient may voice vague complaints, such as, "I'm just not myself lately" or "I don't have the pep I used to have. Can you prescribe a pick-me-up?" Often the patient will say, "I just want to know there is nothing physically wrong with me; it's probably just nerves." One should then inquire about current concerns. You may learn that a relative or friend has recently died or suffered a major illness, prompting the patient to make sure he does not have cancer or some other serious disease.

M.M. is a forty-five-year-old Caucasian school teacher. She has been physically well all her life and has no specific complaint, but she has become concerned about her health status. By asking her to describe a typical day in her life, the clinician discovered that she and her husband are divorcing but still live in the same house. They have hardly spoken for a year and a half and the patient is becoming increasingly tense. She was concerned that the tremendous daily stress was adversely affecting her health.

Other examples of healthy patients requiring continuing care are pregnant women, well-baby visits to a pediatrician, and students who require periodic physical examinations for school purposes. The interview is the vehicle for developing relationships with patients that will help the patient maintain good health behavior.

CARE OF THE PATIENT WITH AN UNCERTAIN DIAGNOSIS

Common complaints for which a specific diagnosis often cannot be made but which call for the continuous care of a patient are fatigue, malaise, lack of energy or "no pep" (but not fatigue), and chronic, non-specific pain. When an illness or health-related problem needs more time to develop before a diagnosis can be made, continuing care is also required. It is very important to be direct with the patient in this situation. State that the diagnosis has not yet been made and that the therapy will be aimed at the symptoms troubling the patient. When appropriate, reassure the patient that the results of the therapy may aid in making the diagnosis. It is most important to direct the interview to the patient's fears and concerns. Support must be given. By specifying the needed follow-up and showing appropriate concern for the patient's worries, the clinician should be able to reassure the patient. It is then much more likely that the latter will adhere to the suggested treatment program.

If the diagnosis remains uncertain, the patient may require increasing support and reassurance. If the patient's life is not significantly affected by the symptoms, he is most likely to accept the uncertainty. If the disruption to his life is great, he will very likely demand more action and more support. It is usually helpful to engage patients in the planning process and give them a sense of control over their own health.

M.S. was a fifty-seven-year-old president of his own manufacturing firm. He required total replacement of both hip joints within the same year. After the second operation, he developed pain in that hip, which persisted for months after the operation. His work required frequent travel and mobility. Because of the disruption to his life caused by the pain, he demanded more action from the physician. The primary physician believed that the pain would eventually diminish or disappear and that it would be a grave error to operate again. With reassurance, judicious use of "expert" outside opinion from consultants, and physical therapy, the patient was given a treatment plan that he felt helped his progress. Equally important was the fact that the patient was allowed to join in the therapy plan by being supported in his desire to seek acupuncture and kinesiology. The result was ultimately successful.

Chronic non-specific pain is another complaint that often results in no specific diagnosis. If the pain is persistent or unrelenting, referral to a pain clinic or specialist may be part of the plan. Patients who feel anxious or depressed perceive pain to a greater extent than those who are not.

Depressed patients, sometimes complaining of fatigue or malaise rather than depression, often need psychiatric consultation. Some of the situations calling for psychiatric consultation are suspected psychotic thought disorder, suspected organic brain syndrome or dementia, and agitation or suicidal behavior. Most commonly, the patient requiring a psychiatric referral is one who has become depressed, anxious, or distraught because of stressful events in his life. Many patients are frightened of psychiatry or are reluctant to admit that they may need psychiatric care. Accordingly, the clinician must approach the subject with delicacy. He should be sensitive to the patient's attitude toward seeing a psychiatrist and his readiness to accept such help. If the patient displays a good deal of resistance to the idea, this should be discussed sufficiently to permit him to get used to the idea.

The patient's initial introduction to the psychiatrist can sometimes be facilitated by a joint visit with the primary care physician. The role of the primary clinician in such a consultation is to validate the patient's complaints and physical symptoms and to help reduce the patient's anxiety. He can clarify the association between the patient's psychological and emotional state and his physical symptoms. Occasional subsequent joint visits throughout the course of treatment may provide valuable support.

E.P. was a thirty-two-year-old surgeon with a history of depression since the age of sixteen. He was in an auto accident and sustained a low back injury. The pain he experienced was aggravated by his depression. He became medically dependent on narcotics and began administering medication to himself. The internist pointed out the role of the depression in his pain problem and suggested a joint session with a psychiatrist in an effort to explore the problem. The patient agreed because the internist accepted the validity of the patient's pain but showed how it related to depression. After the joint consultation, the patient began psychotherapy. With psychotherapy and anti-depressant medication, his depression lifted and he no longer required narcotics.

The use of consultation, whether with a specialist or a diagnostic clinic, can be valuable in the continuing care of a patient with a non-specific diagnosis. If the resulting therapeutic regimen is successful in ameliorating or removing the symptoms, a presumptive diagnosis is made; if the therapy does not work, further plans need to be made. In the first instance, if the presumptive diagnosis is still uncertain, the patient can be reassured that if the symptoms recur, the therapy can be reinstated and further diagnostic studies can be done. In the second case, if the therapeutic plan does not work, continued support is vital. The patient should be reassured that he is not being abandoned. Symptomatic measures should, of course, be continued. Referral to a consultant must be done carefully, so that the patient feels it is a collaborative, supportive move and not one intended to transfer his problem to someone else. For example, the patient with a chronic pain syndrome might be referred to a rheumatologist or pain clinic; a patient with non-specific functional bowel complaints might be referred to a gastro-enterologist. Periodic monitoring of the patient's status by the primary clinician, or even joint visits with the specialist, can add greatly to the patient's sense of well-being. This team approach often gives the patient the feeling that the physicians are following his illness closely even if the diagnosis remains elusive.

THE PATIENT WITH A CHRONIC DISEASE

The practice of a primary care practitioner largely consists of patients with chronic diseases, such as arthritis, diabetes, chronic obstructive pulmonary disease, and cardiovascular disease. Such chronic illness is an ever-present part of the patient's existence, so it is important to assess its impact. This includes changes in activities and pursuits caused by the disease, the area of lost function, as well as social and economic aspects. The psychological

effects of any impairment may be lessened if there are helpful re-
sources available to the patient, such as family, friends, and colleagues. If the patient has dealt successfully with past reverses, he
will predictably adjust to a disability more easily.

For example, a progressive muscular dystrophy may advance
from only slight atrophy and good mobility to marked muscle
wasting and confinement to a wheelchair or bed. Successful functioning within the limits imposed by the disease will be directly
related to the patient's sense of hope and his motivation to be active. If the patient feels the clinician is his ally and recognizes the
degree of loss caused by the illness, he is much more likely to cooperate with rehabilitation efforts. Thus, enthusiastic participation
in physical therapy programs, achievement of realistic (even if limited) rehabilitation goals, and maximal utilization of available re-
sources can be greatly facilitated by the clinician who is a skillful
interviewer.

> An attractive thirty-seven-year-old woman with autosomal dominant
> muscular dystrophy progressed over a seven-year period from being a
> dancer to walking only with the aid of braces and crutches. The
> limitations imposed by the illness were severe in that her self-esteem
> was largely based on her attractiveness and her dancing. Interviewing
> brought out the fact that she had never been successful in establishing
> lasting relationships with men. She was a gregarious person and very
> ambitious. Her father died in a wheelchair, and many cousins have
> the illness at different stages, though her sister does not.

Helping this patient to express her feelings about her father and
her sister and about the loss of her dancing ability is clearly an
essential part of the interview. How she compares herself to other
members of the family with the illness, how she views herself
sexually before and after the disability, and how she has dealt with
men are all important concerns for the clinician if he is to be
maximally helpful. Helping the patient to express these concerns
and feelings and providing support helps reduce their intensity.
One need not feel that this must be done in one interview.

continuing care of such patients provides opportunities for the clinician to deal with the patient's feelings repeatedly.

> F.L., a sixty-year-old lawyer, was diagnosed as having diabetes of adult onset ten years earlier. He now requires insulin. Both his father and brother had diabetes and both died of heart attacks in their sixties. He was still working since work was a major part of his life, yet he wondered if he should retire. Being divorced, his social life largely revolved around eating in restaurants. He had cataracts, which were progressing rapidly now, and could no longer drive at night. He was fearful of the future and pessimistic about living much longer, though there was no evidence of coronary disease. The clinician helped him to express his fear of death after he expressed his feelings about his father and brother. It was then possible to give him reassurance that he did not have coronary disease.

Chronic illness almost invariably impairs the quality of a patient's life. Improving it may depend on the clinician's use of his art, for medical science often has little to offer in the way of definitive treatment. These patients usually experience anger, frustration, depression, and anxiety, with a consequent fatigue and loss of energy. The empathic clinician facilitates the expression of the patient's feelings. Since the illness will usually progress, a tactful discussion of the prognosis, as far as the patient is capable of accepting it, can help relieve anxiety and depression. One should choose the time for such discussion with care. When a patient is demoralized, only support should be given.

TH⸱   PATIENT

⸱ the care of patients with fatal illness who are still
⸱nal is to help maintain the quality of their re-
⸱tever degree possible. In part, this is promoted
⸱setting realistic goals. One aspect is helping
⸱rs in order." Questions often raised by pa-

1. Am I able to travel? (e.g., overseas or locally to visit relatives)
2. Can I continue to work?
3. How should I plan for my children?

The physician should then assess the importance of such travel or continued work for each patient. This must be weighed against their ability to endure travel or work. Some patients are relieved to be able to stop working; others feel lost without it. Some patients will need to be reminded to make a will or get financial counseling. Discreet inquiries into these matters and advice, when appropriate, can aid a patient in achieving realistic goals before his death.

> R.B., a fifty-four-year-old bartender, had just been told he had squamous cell carcinoma of the mouth. He came to see the physician because of a lump on his neck of one month's duration. He told his physician, "I want you to tell me if I have nothing to worry about." He had been taking a friend to radiation therapy for treatment of metastatic cancer. R.B. had previously been seen regularly because of alcoholism and inflammatory bowel disease, both of which were in remission. He had missed his last appointment when the lump first appeared. This interview occurred shortly after he reported the lump to his physician.

> DOCTOR: The biopsy shows that you have a tumor in your mouth.
> PATIENT: Jesus, doc, I can't believe it. Is it malignant?
> DOCTOR: Yes.
> PATIENT: So come on, doc, say it. Does that mean I have . . .
> DOCTOR: You have cancer.
> PATIENT: Oh, Christ (*looking down and shaking his head*). It can't be. I was just getting well and now this. Well, what do my chances look like—better than 75 per cent?
> DOCTOR: Well, Dick, it's too early to tell yet, but it does not appear to have spread beyond your neck. The usual treatment for something like this is surgery. The surgery is uncomfortable but not hazardous, and then you will have radiation therapy for six weeks after surgery. With good results from that, and with no evidence of spread, the radiation therapy should help a good deal.

PATIENT: Well, two years ago you thought I would die, and I made it through that surgery. I'll make it through this one. (*After a moment of silence*) But, look, is this one different? Should I make sure Ann is taken care of before the operation?

The patient's initial reaction to learning of his diagnosis was fear and denial. He tried to set a limit on how much information he wanted. He did not want to know of less than a 75 per cent chance of survival. Yet he needed the reassurance that he need not set his affairs in order at once, that he would not be leaving his wife uncared for if he didn't. By telling him the surgery is not hazardous and radiation therapy can help, the clinician is reassuring the patient that the diagnosis of cancer does not imply immediate death. At this point, that was all that was necessary.

When cancer recurs after having been treated, the response is somewhat different. Patients must now cope with the news that the treatment was not successful. They will usually experience a more serious reactive depression than when the original diagnosis was reported. They must now adjust to increasing dependence on others, to a decline in job and family roles, and to changes in relationships with others. At this time, too, patients must face death in a more immediate sense, and feelings of hopelessness and finality are much more intense.[1]

As death approaches, one can expect a series of changes in the patient's attitude toward himself, the world, and dying itself. Kubler-Ross[2] described the responses of over two hundred patients at the University of Chicago Billings Hospital in terms of five stages: denial and isolation; anger; bargaining; depression; and acceptance. However, most clinicians who work with dying patients have not found these five stages occurring in all patients, nor in any particular order. Patients may not experience some of them, may move back and forth between them, and do not necessarily achieve acceptance before they die. Patients must cope with loss of dignity. To reinforce their efforts to maintain dignity and self-respect, one must help them cope with their fears, and this requires a supportive attitude.

G.S., a sixty-three-year-old actor, had metastatic cancer of the pancreas. He was mobile but had to wear a nasogastric tube, through which he received a liquid diet. He required intermittent suction to relieve nausea and to prevent distention and vomiting. At the time of this interview, he knew he was dying but was not yet terminal. During the course of the interview, the doctor was able to facilitate expression of his feelings about dying.

PATIENT: I love my wife and my friends. I have had a very full life, and I do not wish to leave them (*tears begin*). I do not want to die, doctor, and I'm angry at the lack of help your profession affords me.

DOCTOR: What would you like from your doctors?

PATIENT: I would like to be cured, to go on unrestrictedly with my life, sharing each day with my wife and the people who love me. But I do not expect this (*eyes and face are lowered*). I'm forced to accept that this is the final act in my play.

DOCTOR: What would you like from me?

PATIENT: I have three requests: that I die without pain; that I die with dignity and remain in control of my bodily functions; and that I remain mentally alert. If you can accomplish this, if you can do this, you will have fulfilled your Hippocratic Oath.

DOCTOR: I will do my best.

The patient had outlined his goals for the terminal stage of his life. He was angry and depressed, the anger being displaced to the clinician. His need for a nasogastric tube reduced his sense of dignity. By enabling the patient to unburden himself, the clinician helped him set goals for the last part of his life. Remaining pain-free and maintaining control of bodily functions may not be possible in the terminal stages of cancer, but G. S. did achieve his goals even though he remained angry and depressed until his death. All patients do not achieve acceptance of death, and the clinician should be prepared for this eventuality.

Whatever form the dying patient's experience may take, he will surely require support. This should, in turn, make it easier for him to deal as honestly with himself and his loved ones as possible. Each patient has unique needs to meet at the time of his death.

By allowing patients to express and share their anger, denial, depression, and fear, the clinician helps them find the energy to meet their personal needs before they die. Open-ended interviewing permits patients to deal with their feelings about death at a pace they can tolerate.

With adults, the clinician should work toward an understanding of the situation at the rate chosen by the patient. This means answering questions honestly and making time available to patients so that they may talk about their feelings and ask whatever questions they may have. One should never force information on patients that they are not yet able to accept. If a patient never gets beyond denial, the clinician should not view this as a failure but simply as the limit of what this patient could accept.

A knowledge of the patient's psychological and emotional makeup is essential in deciding what information to provide and how to deliver it. The patient who denies that he is fatally ill must be permitted to accept the facts slowly; if he cannot, he should be permitted to deny them. The cool, objective, somewhat compulsive person may ask for a detailed scientific explanation. This should be given. Others want to know the bare minimum, and no more. This, too, should be respected. To choose the right approach, one must know the patient.

Likewise, the clinician needs to be fairly comfortable with his own feelings about death so that he can allow the patient to share his deepest feelings. The clinician should not try to mask his emotional response to the patient's expression of feeling. While the experience can be draining to both patient and doctor, the shared vulnerability can be rewarding to both, and can add to the clinician's understanding of patients at the end of life.

Clinicians who work with cancer patients for many years often report that although they began by being supportive and getting personally involved with their cancer patients, they eventually found this to be too heavy an emotional burden and increasingly tried to keep their distance. This is sometimes referred to as "burn-out." It requires that the physicians, nurses, and other health professionals who work with cancer patients be given the opportunity to share their feelings and find support for the stress their work places upon them.

REFERENCES

1. Abrams, R. D., "The Patient with Cancer: His Changing Pattern of Communication," *New England Journal of Medicine*, 274:317-322, 1966.
2. Kubler-Ross, E., *On Death and Dying*. New York: The Macmillan Company, 1969.

INDEX